FAST
AFTER
50

FAST AFTER 50

HOW TO RACE STRONG
FOR THE REST OF YOUR LIFE

JOE FRIEL

VELO press

Boulder, Colorado

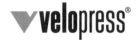

3002 Sterling Circle, Suite 100
Boulder, Colorado 80301-2338 USA
(303) 440-0601 · Fax (303) 444-6788 · E-mail velopress@competitorgroup.com

Distributed in the United States and Canada by Ingram Publisher Services

A Cataloging-in-Publication record for this book is available from the Library of Congress.
ISBN 978-1-937715-26-7

For information on purchasing VeloPress books, please call (800) 811-4210, ext. 2138, or visit www.velopress.com.

This paper meets the requirements of ANSI/NISO Z39.48-1992 (Permanence of Paper).

Cover design by Kevin Roberson
Cover illustration by Alex Williamson
Cover photograph by Philip Beckman
Back cover photograph by Dan Watson/The Signal Newspaper
Interior design by Vicki Hopewell

Text set in Sackers Gothic, Titillium, and Mercury

15   16   17 / 10   9   8   7   6   5   4   3   2

For all of the older athletes I've known and coached.
Thank you for being role models and teachers
for so many younger athletes.

CONTENTS

Prologue

I'm 70.

There. I've said it.

That dreaded birthday arrived shortly after I started writing this book. None of my previous many-candle birthdays—40, 50, or even 60—got my attention. But 70 did. Somehow, 70 seems really old, a *lot* older than 69. It seemed different enough to me that I had been contemplating the start of my eighth decade of life for the better part of a year. My greatest concern was that it might signal the beginning of the end of my lifelong adventure as a serious athlete. I simply didn't know what to expect.

Six months prior to the Big Day, I decided to do something about it. I was going to read all of the aging research I could find to see if I could determine my future as an old athlete. I also wanted to learn what I could do to avoid a big decline in performance. The last time I read the aging research was in the mid-1990s when I wrote a book titled *Cycling Past 50*. I was 53 at the time. There wasn't much research on aging available back then. But with the huge baby-boom generation entering their 60s starting in 2005 and the impact of their arrival en masse on American life, I found that this picture had changed considerably.

In the past 15 years or so, a tremendous amount of research on aging had been done. I read those studies almost daily for the better part of a year. I started seeing interesting patterns in them. And so in the late summer of 2013, only a few months into the project, I decided to write a blog about what I was learning. That turned into 29 posts (www.joefrielsblog .com) on the topic of aging, which drew a great deal of positive feedback from readers. The tremendous response from older athletes convinced me that I needed to write a book on the topic to reach a bigger audience and tell them what I had learned. As it turned out, my publisher, Velo-Press, had been looking for someone to write such a book.

You now have in your hands my personal birthday present for all senior athletes. I hope it helps you answer your questions about aging, which I am sure are the same questions that I had at the start of the project. Of course, there's only one question we all want the answer to, the same one I pondered prior to my Big Seven-Zero Day: How can I slow, or perhaps even temporarily reverse, the loss of performance as I get older?

By the time we're in our 50s, it's just starting to become apparent that things are going the wrong way. The first thing athletes typically notice around that age is that they don't recover from a race or a hard training session as quickly as they did a few years earlier. And not only that—race times are slowing, there's a loss of power, hills seem steeper, and other performance markers are also looking worse. What can be done?

My purpose in writing this book is to help you answer that question by coming to understand what sport science says about the senior athlete's performance, training, and lifestyle. If you've already thumbed through the pages, you've probably noticed two things: There are lots of numbered notes in the text, and they lead to scientific sources that are collected by chapter at the end of the book. You may not be used to reading books like this. At first glance, this level of source citation may make the book look more like a college textbook than an entertaining read. But I've included those notes and references for a reason. I believe it is necessary to provide some degree of proof about what I am proposing you do in your training to improve performance, rather than just offering unvalidated opinions.

There are two basic sources of information about aging: research and opinion. Both are valuable in some way. When it comes to the value of opinion, it depends on the source. Is the source knowledgeable and experienced with a long history of working with aging athletes and endurance sports? Does the opinion come from someone who also is an aging athlete? Or are you reading the opinion of someone who has very little background in sport, knows little about physiology, and is talking off the top of his or her head with nothing to back it up? I highly value the opinions of a few known, learned people, but pay little attention to the ramblings of most on this and related topics. Too much of what we hear about aging is based on hearsay and old wives' tales. Older athletes' thoughts on the topic can be insightful but are subject to unique situations that may or may not be applicable to others.

On the other hand, I place a high value on the thoughts of those with a scientific slant to their understanding of the world. They ask hard questions and seek answers regardless of what ideas may be popular. If their opinions are also based on research studies that control most all of the things that can influence the outcomes and are published in peer-reviewed journals, all the better. I've always relied heavily on science to help shape my opinions when it comes to training. That's especially valuable with topics such as aging and sport performance since there have been so few older athletes preceding the boomer generation whom we could rely on for answers. I also didn't want to simply give you my opinions on such an important topic without some solid evidence to back them up. That's why you see all of the references in my notes.

All of this doesn't mean my opinions aren't included. They most certainly are, as the research studies still need to be interpreted and applied to real life. What you will read in the following chapters, therefore, are my opinions on aging as shaped by the research.

If you also need to understand why things are the way they are, you can trace the origins of my opinions by finding the sources in the notes at the end of the book and doing a quick search for each one online. The best source of research abstracts (a brief summary of a study) can be found online at PubMed. This website (http://www.ncbi.nlm.nih.gov/pubmed) is owned and operated by the U.S. government's National Center for Biotechnology Information, a division of the National Institutes of Health. Once you've found a study's abstract, you can learn even more about the topic by chasing down the related research studies listed on the right side of the page. Most readers will probably find this tedious and unnecessary. If so, you can simply ignore the notes and references. But the option is there should you want to know more about some topic or see how I came to my conclusions.

I hope you don't take this to mean that science knows everything about aging and how you should train and live your life in order to perform at a high level. It certainly doesn't. The best we can hope for is to be pointed in the right direction. Sport science has an especially poor record when it comes to paving new pathways in sport. It has nearly always lagged behind most of the important changes that happen.

For example, sport science didn't come up with the Fosbury Flop high-jump technique. It was conceived and first used in the 1960s by Dick Fosbury, a college athlete, not a scientist. But later on, after high-jump records started falling because of this new technique, science explained why it was so much more effective than the eastern roll, western roll, and straddle methods that had been used for the better part of a century. (The key is that with the Flop technique, the jumper's center of gravity passes under the bar rather than over it.) Now all world-class high jumpers do the Flop.

Sport science also didn't invent aerodynamic handlebars for the bicycle. They were the brainchild of a Montana ski coach turned cycling enthusiast by the name of Boone Lennon. Sport science later reported on why they work so well (they greatly reduce drag caused by the body, which is the greatest impediment to going fast on a bike). If you're a triathlete or road cyclist who does time trials, you know all about this. The list of things sport science figured out after the fact could go on and on. It's rare for science to lead the way on anything substantial in sport.

There are useful exceptions, however. Training periodization, which nearly all serious athletes use to design their seasons, originated from sport scientists in the Eastern bloc countries in the early 20th century and continues to be refined by scientists to this day. A good example of recent development comes from sport scientist Vladimer Issurin, who is largely credited with coming up with a highly focused training method called "Block Periodization" that is used by many elite athletes. More recently we've seen the development of training concepts, technology, and related analysis tools from sport scientists such as Eric Banister, David Costill, Tim Noakes, and Andrew Coggan.

Of course, many scientists these days are also athletes. Their and many others' contributions to sport have had a significant impact on how athletes train. But such breakthroughs in training aren't common. It's largely athletes and coaches, not scientists, who do the innovating.

To further confound the matter, what research there is on many aspects of lifestyle and sport performance has not been done using older athletes as subjects. So we have to decide whether studies using young subjects are applicable to us as senior athletes. Even worse, the subjects in these studies are often not athletes, and they are seldom women. Men make up by far the greatest portion of the subjects in studies on aging as well as nearly all other sports-related topics. Scientists used to think that men and women were the same in all areas of study that weren't directly related to gender, such as menopause. But that's now changing as many scientists begin to realize that women differ from men in subtle ways. Hence, there is a growing but still small body of research dedicated to men- or women-only subjects. All of this means that even though there may be research on a given topic, it may not match our unique needs as senior athletes.

And so we come back to performance with aging and how athletes and scientists are revising the way we think about growing old. Defining the "aging athlete" is difficult, especially in the conventional way with a number representing age. Yet with each new number comes change. We know that change will happen with aging; we just don't know how rapidly it will occur. Some athletes continue to produce amazing performances well into their later years and remain competitive even with other athletes half their age. Locally they are thought of as legends and are held in high regard by younger athletes. Others with the same number of birthdays appear to age quickly and see significant drops in performance. Why the difference? How is it that some seem to have found the fountain of youth while others have missed it? Genetics can probably explain much of this, but not all as you'll read in the following pages. Some older athletes have also discovered what it takes in training and lifestyle to keep performance decreases from reflecting aging increases.

For example, consider the remarkable accomplishment of Diana Nyad, who in 2013 swam from Cuba to Florida—111 miles and nearly 53 nonstop hours in shark- and jellyfish-infested rough water—at age 64. She obviously knows something about aging, performance, and especially motivation. I'm sure you've read of her accomplishment. But she isn't the only aging athlete turning in amazing performances. We haven't learned of most of the others as their stories rarely make the front page. Hundreds of aging athletes achieve exceptional sport feats that most of us never hear of. One is Bob Scott.

At age 75, racing in the Ironman® World Championship in Hawaii, Bob Scott set a new course record of 13:27:50 for his age group. That's a good time even for athletes in their 30s and 40s. Winning and breaking triathlon records is nothing new for him. Four years earlier, he set the men's 70–74 age-group record at 12:59:02, finishing more than 90 minutes ahead of the second age-group finisher. If the sport of triathlon supplied a list of age-adjusted race winners, Bob would nearly always take the gold medal.

Or how about Libby James, age 76, of Fort Collins, Colorado? She set a new half-marathon world record of 1:45:56 for her age category in 2013, demolishing the previous record of 1:55:19. Few women half her age can run such a fast time. As it happens, running does provide age-graded results, and Libby's record time topped all other half marathoners for that year regardless of age or gender.

A list of such amazing accomplishments from aging athletes could go on and on. You may never swim from Cuba to Florida or break course or world records, but I expect you are capable of achieving far more than you are currently accomplishing. How can you do it? How can you be fast after 50? That's what I hope you will learn by reading this book.

The book is arranged in two parts. Part I, Chapters 1 through 3, will describe the many challenges facing the aging athlete. In Part II, Chapters 4 through 8, I propose solutions to those problems. These involve not only training solutions but also those that we consider to be part of the way we live—our lifestyle. The two really can't be separated.

How about the title: Fast After 50? Will you become "fast" by applying what you learn here? The answer depends on many variables: how well you've trained in the past few years, how motivated you are, how willing you are to make changes, how many confounding factors such as health concerns you have, and much more. As I am sure you have learned over the years, there are no automatic fixes for performance. There are only dedication and discipline when it comes to change. But I can guarantee that if you keep doing what you've been doing, you'll keep getting the same results—or worse. With aging, change is necessary.

What should you change? The answer depends on what may be holding you back from once again becoming fast. According to the research, the list is most likely to include decreasing aerobic capacity, increasing body fat, and shrinking muscles. Those three problems and their solutions are what this book is all about.

The solutions, described in detail in Part II, are high-intensity training, including intervals and heavy-load strength work; periodization changes; and lifestyle modification involving sleep, nutrition, and training recovery methods. Along the way you will learn more about how your aging body operates and the details of gently coaxing it to greater fitness despite your age. That's the book in a nutshell.

The solutions I'm going to suggest are probably contrary to much of what you've been told. The long-held traditional advice from the medical community has been that older people (usually meaning age 50 and over) should avoid strenuous exercise. It's dangerous, they tell us. You're likely to die if you're not seriously injured first. Instead of searching for performance gains, once we reach that doddering age we should walk—not too fast, mind you; work in the garden; and, at most, square dance on occasion or participate in water aerobics classes.

I suspect that since you're reading this book you don't subscribe to such advice. Your parents may have, but not you. That doesn't mean you have no concerns when it comes to vigorous exercise. I have them, too. So I'll try to help you make decisions along the way about how great the changes should be, how quickly they may be incorporated into your life and training, and what to watch out for along the way.

Let's get started down the path to better sport performance regardless of age.

PART I

OLDER
SLOWER
FATTER?

We've been told that as we age, we can expect a rapid decline in physical attributes, especially those that determine performance in endurance sports. There are many questions we athletes typically have about this topic: Are the changes inevitable? How rapidly can we expect the changes to occur? What is the cause of the changes? Can we do anything to slow or stop the decline? Is it possible to reverse the changes? You've probably pondered some of these as you've gotten older. In Chapters 1 through 3, we will seek the answers.

THE AGING MYTH

Aging is not lost youth, but a new stage of opportunity and strength.

—BETTY FRIEDAN

What can you expect to happen to your body in the next 10, 20, 30 years? You've seen others grow old but never thought it would happen to you. You're an athlete. You've kept yourself in good shape. You may not even remember the last time you caught a cold. Sure, you've probably collected a few injuries over the years, but what athlete hasn't? Fitness and competition have always been a big part of your life. Can't things stay that way?

There may be plenty of voices telling you that you shouldn't be exercising so strenuously, that advancing age means you *must* slow down. Maybe they're telling you horror stories of broken bones and heart attacks. *Look at so-and-so,* they say. *He wouldn't stop, and now he's getting knee replacements. Quit training and competing. Overdoing it is bad for you. No one keeps racing forever. Back off—you've earned a rest. Enjoy the twilight of your life.*

Of course you wouldn't be reading this book if you bought into such antiquated notions about life and exercise. And rest assured that you can indeed remain vigorous well into your 50s, 60s, 70s, and beyond. By "vigorous," I mean fully capable of training hard and producing high-quality performances in your sport.

What does it take to do that? Is it possible to slow or even reverse the aging process to stay fast—or even get faster—in the coming years? Yes, it is. I hope you believe it is because that's where we're headed in this book. I'll show you how others do it and how you can do it, too.

The journey may turn out to be an emotional roller coaster for you. I'm not going to pull any punches. You must be prepared to give full consideration to many matters—that is, if you truly want to be fast after 50, 60, 70, or whatever your age may be. But if you've been an athlete all your life, and if competition is a big part of who you are, you already know how to work hard to reach high goals. If you have that kind of determination, you can do it.

But let's not get ahead of ourselves. First things first. We need to start at the beginning.

What Is Aging?

From an athlete's perspective, what is aging all about? Perhaps we should start by giving old age a personal point of view.

Remember how old and feeble your grandparents seemed when you were a youngster? And what about your parents? They probably were ancient in your mind when you were a teenager, but looking back now, you realize they really weren't. They were still young and vibrant then— just kids. Over the next few decades, you watched them morph into old age. That also left an impression on you of what becoming old means. In your head there's a folder titled "Old Age" in which you have filed some

Body Learning:
The Athletic Fountain of Youth

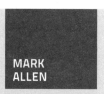

MARK
ALLEN

I'm 56 years old. I'm a six-time Hawaii Ironman World Champion. I'm 20 years out from my final title in 1995. I don't swim, bike, and run for a living anymore. But I do exercise about 350 days a year, and at least 300 of those days include a surfing session at one of my local breaks here in Santa Cruz, California. Interestingly, I have recently taken that sport to a whole new personal level, gaining flow, power, and that final bit extra I've been searching for—from each bottom turn, every snap off the top and tube ride—but which had eluded me since I started surfing as a teenager nearly 40 years ago.

I'm not telling you this to brag but as a personal living testament of the potential we all have in athletics as we age. I should not be surfing my life's best at age 56, but I am! Why? There are a few reasons.

The first is consistency in training. Regardless of your sport and regardless of your age, consistently doing your sport is what builds expertise and carries that improvement curve on long into the future. What I mean by "consistency" is not just doing the same thing over and over in the same way. I mean that you consistently make a commitment to refine the mechanics of how your body moves in all the required motions of your sport. I mean you make it your goal to have your body learn something new each and every day that you train.

Athletes who train without focusing on learning wear down. They get injured. They become rigid and less efficient as they age. They can also get frustrated. Without a commitment to body learning, it's tough to keep any sport fresh, to keep outdistancing your age by gaining new levels of performance. However, those who continually search for more flow and fluidity, more power within the range of motion required of them, athletes who continually work just that small bit beyond what is required on race day, end up getting faster and better even into their »

Continued

later years. The key mind-set is a dedication to learning something new from the ground floor up every single time you go out and do your sport.

Here's how it works for me in the ocean. First, surfing obviously requires conditioning (cardiovascular, muscular strength, endurance for paddling, flexibility for bending and twisting in all directions). Clearly, I have a lot of the cardio and endurance from my years as a triathlete, but I continue to run to keep the ticker strong, and I do heaps of dry-land, full-range-of-motion functional strength work to keep every muscle healthy and strong yet loose. All of this is focused not only on improving performance but also on preventing injury, which for an aging athlete can be a death sentence. That is actually my top priority: to prevent injury so that I can be consistent in my sport.

Second, I watch how the best move. How do they surf? Where are they on the wave? Where on the wave do they make their turns? I look to see how they manage to pull into a tube that seems to appear out of nowhere. Then it's my turn. I pick one aspect to perfect. Maybe it's my bottom turn; perhaps it's a cutback. Whatever it is, I pick one element that I'm going to focus on over and over on each wave until I start to feel that it's happening without any effort or thinking on my part. I then continue to work on it until it starts to take on a dynamic quality that feels like how the best in the sport look. I know I don't look like them, but I can feel like them! I did this as a triathlete. I watched the best cyclists, the best runners in the world, and I imprinted in my mind how they moved. Then I made it my commitment to try to have that same feel in my movements. That commitment paid off with dramatic improvements in performance even though I was doing absolutely no more actual training.

Perfect one area at a time until it becomes a new level of automatic movement. That's body learning. It takes me about a full year to really gain what I am looking for from each part of my surfing. I shifted into » this mind-set of body learning when I turned 50 because I could see that my surfing was more or less the same as it had been for the bulk of my life. I wanted to try a new approach to see if I could actually improve, even though I was clearly aging.

Year one of this focus was devoted to getting in the tube and actually making it back out on a consistent basis. Year two was working on the takeoff, being able to get into the wave smoothly in a lot of different conditions and sizes. Year three was refining the bottom turn, exploding off it with just the right trajectory to set me where I wanted to be in the face of the wave standing up in front of me. Year four was the cutback, being able to turn back into the most critical part of the wave. Year five was snapping off the top and then back down the face to control speed and meet the wave at its most dramatic upright position.

Year six (this year), it all came together. Each element was there at the exact moment it was called for by the dynamic of the wave at hand. No thought, no struggle, just a flow that tied together a few thousand hours of a mind-set that took learning from the ground floor up and brought it all together wave after wave—at age 56!

Having my body keep learning has been as critical to athletic performance and overall suppleness as the actual exercise where the learning takes place. It really is the athletic fountain of youth!

defining documents based on your experiences growing up. Your grandparents and parents are in it, along with some of your friends who have definitely become old right in front of your eyes. "That won't happen to me," you've told yourself. And it probably hasn't, because you've stayed active. They haven't.

You can almost certainly find signs, however, that your body is changing. You obviously aren't a kid anymore. You don't get carded when you order a beer. People treat you with a bit more respect than when you were young. They call you "Mr." or "Mrs." They see something about you now that says "old." Maybe it's your graying hair and the faint wrinkles starting to show in your face. Or perhaps it's the tightness in your back that is apparent when you stand up a little more slowly than you used to. It doesn't matter. You know you can still whup most of them in your sport. They know it, too, and have a lot of respect for you because of how you're redefining aging for them. You've become a role model for many younger people, and it's apparent.

Do you have any grandchildren? That can be a real game-changer. It has been for me. Apparently my choices in clothes ("Funny shirt, Grampy!") and music ("Who are the Beatles?") send a strong message to my 11-year-old granddaughter. Of course, if you're like me, you don't see anything wrong with either your clothes, your music, or anything else. It's just you.

None of this alters the fact that you're seeing physical changes, probably more than mental changes, although those may be popping up more often now, too. What's causing all of this to happen to you, and what can you expect in the coming years? Science has been addressing that question for decades. How about your athletic performance? You are undoubtedly aware of changes there. Are they normal? Perhaps you know athletes older than you who are well known for their continued athleticism. What do they do that sets them apart? Can you replicate it? Can you train and compete at a higher level of performance than you are currently doing? And can you keep doing so into the future? That's a huge challenge. But I'm certain it's possible. I've seen it happen with other athletes.

It boils down to the choices you make every day of your life. These choices are not just about training but include every lifestyle decision, big or small. All are important. In this book we'll primarily examine those that are specific to sport performance. But don't think it ends there. There is much more to slowing the aging process than training. We'll take a look at ways to fight back in Chapter 2.

"Normal" Aging

How does science explain the phenomenon we call "aging"? Interestingly, scientists are still working on that question. They don't fully understand it yet. They have theories, and there is ongoing research, but they don't have solid answers. Instead, most researchers have chosen to examine only the symptoms of growing older. Looking at symptoms is easier, so there has been a ton of such research over the past few decades as the average age of our population continues to rise.

So what does science say we should expect from aging? What are those dreaded symptoms? Here's a partial shopping list of run-of-the-mill signs of aging as reported in most of the research:

- Skin loses its elasticity and becomes drier as oil glands slow their production. Fingernails grow more slowly.
- Hair thins, and there's more gray hair as pigment cells are reduced.
- Compression of joints, including spinal discs, causes a loss of height. By age 80, the loss of 2 inches is common.
- Somewhere around age 55, high-frequency sounds start becoming harder to hear.
- By age 50, most people need reading glasses as the eyes' lenses become less flexible, impairing the ability to focus on anything close up.
- Changes occur in the menstrual cycle before it ceases.
- Sleep time typically becomes shorter, and the quality of sleep decreases. Waking often during the night is common.

- Bone minerals are lost, resulting in more fragility.
- The basic metabolic rate slows down, often resulting in weight gain—mostly fat.

Obvious stuff. Nothing really new here. You're probably personally aware of at least some of these symptoms, and this is just the short list. We could go on by looking at what happens to the brain, nervous system, heart, blood vessels, lungs, kidneys, urinary system, and sexual function. Additionally, and sadly, the chances of contracting ailments such as osteoarthritis, hypothyroidism, type 2 diabetes, high blood pressure, cancer, coronary artery disease, Alzheimer's disease, Parkinson's disease, and dementia increase. All of this is what the folks in the white lab coats tell us and have been saying for decades. According to them, none of us would want the symptoms of physical aging. Let me off this train!

There's a caveat, however. It's important for you to understand that what we know of all these depressing changes has been based on studies of *normal* aging people. By "normal" I mean people who are generally representative of our society—many of whom are sedentary, overweight, and unmotivated. Even at a young age, most normal folks are already experiencing the early stages of some of these symptoms, and they are taking pills to ward off the worst of them. Exercise and nutrition aren't part of the program as far as normal people are concerned.

Since these people make up the bulk of society, they are considered to be common markers of the state of human physiology—in a word, *normal*. But they certainly aren't normal for our human genus or the entire *Homo sapiens* species. Instead, these types are unhealthy, and they simply don't know it. They believe what's happening to them is inevitable, and they may believe they have no control over it. The best they can hope for is that a new pill may come along. The worst of it is that our society has come to accept this as a normal view of aging and even promotes it to the masses.

We didn't evolve for more than two million years to sit in front of a TV eating potato chips and contracting lifestyle diseases. Humans were meant to be active, to move vigorously and strenuously—just as you do as an athlete. Our prehistoric ancestors did that for eons. They really had no choice. Fitness was a condition of survival. They were athletes in the broadest sense of the word. They certainly weren't couch potatoes. Contrary to popular belief, many lived well into their 50s and 60s and beyond.[1] The "died young" idea—the notion that previous generations didn't live nearly as long as we hope to— is based on average life expectancy of the entire population, which was low because so many infants died. If our ancestors survived infancy, though, strenuous activity and a diet devoid of junk food kept them healthy for many decades.

HUMANS WERE meant to be active, to move vigorously and strenuously—just as you do as an athlete.

Much of what science "knows" about the indicators of aging probably doesn't apply to you. You are much less likely than your "normal" neighbor to contract the lifestyle diseases of aging. You aren't normal—*and that's good.* You are continuing the active and vigorous lifestyle of our ancestors. You're an athlete.

As an aging athlete, you are still experiencing some markers of aging, but from a smaller subset of symptoms. Even sedentary people experience these, but they aren't aware of them due to their lack of vigor. For an athlete, however, they stand out—and they are paramount because they have to do with performance. Nearly all exercise physiology research has found that you can expect certain performance-diminishing changes with advancing age. These are the symptoms we need to reverse or at least minimize in our training and lifestyle, and they are the ones we will thoroughly investigate in the coming chapters.

The symptoms of aging that concern athletes include:

- Aerobic capacity (VO_2max) declines.
- Maximal heart rate is reduced.
- The volume of blood pumped with each heartbeat decreases.
- Muscle fibers are lost, resulting in decreased muscle mass and less strength.
- Aerobic enzymes in the muscles become less effective and abundant.
- Blood volume is reduced.

There's more, although these are enough to make you want to avoid birthday parties. But take heart—not all of the research agrees on these symptoms of aging. We'll explore this confusion and what it means for us in later chapters.

Nevertheless, you are undoubtedly experiencing at least some of these common athletic aging markers now. And the older you are, the more aware of them you are. Can anything be done to delay, reduce, or even reverse the negative changes? Yes, it can. Those answers also come from the scientific literature. In Part II we'll take a look at solutions for these performance-related vagaries. Before getting into all of that, however, it's important to understand the impact of these physiological symptoms of aging on your endurance performance.

Performance and Aging

Rather than comparing ourselves with normal people, we'll gain more insight into our needs by seeing what active, fit, and highly motivated older humans are capable of doing. There aren't as many of these people—after all, they aren't normal—but they often reveal what is possible at the highest levels of athletic performance. Here is a quick summary of what we know about the very best endurance athletes' performances relative to age.

In the young athlete's teens and early 20s, physical performance improves rapidly for about 10 years. Around age 30, plus or minus 5 years (it depends on the sport), there is typically a peak in performance. Following that peak, there is a slow decline year after year. This physiological decline can be masked by other changes, many of which can be attributed to experience: As you learn more about how to train and race, performance gains are still possible, if not at the same rate as before. But the decline eventually becomes apparent.

At first, the drop-off for the 30-something athlete just past his or her prime is so slight that it may not even be noticed. In fact, it may be attributed to poor training, minor changes in lifestyle, or even bad luck. But by the early 40s, it is generally obvious to most high-performance athletes that things are going the wrong direction. Professional athletes in their 40s are not common, but there are some. In our realm of endurance sports, Chris Horner, who at age 41 won the Vuelta a España, Spain's three-week bicycle race, is a recent example.

After age 40, the downward trend continues, and by the mid-40s, there are no more professional athletes in the most popular endurance sports. What we're interested in, of course, is the performance trend in the later decades of life, well beyond 40-something. I'm sure you know from experience that the real decline shows up a few years later. So let's look there.

By examining age-group performances in endurance sports, we can get a good idea of what older athletes are capable of doing. This is where the scientific research on symptoms comes in. The problem with many studies of athletes and aging, however, is that they look at broad cross-sections of various age categories by gender. That means they are comparing a wide range of abilities—from the front of the pack to the back—with not only physiology but also motivation playing a huge role in performance. Some people simply aren't motivated to train and don't push themselves anywhere near their limits in a race.

As the number of participants in endurance sports increases (which it has for the past 30 years or so), the percentage of those who are not really concerned about performance and are racing only for social reasons is likely to increase as well. That increase dilutes the data, making it difficult to know what the true impact of age on performance is likely to be just by looking at all age results.

WE'LL GAIN INSIGHT into our needs by seeing what active, fit, and highly motivated older humans are capable of doing.

By looking instead at the race results of world- and national-class age-group athletes, we can get a much better indicator of the limits of human performance and how rapidly the decline in performance occurs with aging. One way of doing that is to examine what the best of the best—the most fit of the aging population—are capable of doing in common endurance sports. That means examining world and national record holders in timed endurance competitions. Does aging still take a huge bite out of their performance? Let's take a look. Seeing what the very best of your age and gender peers are accomplishing, perhaps even in your own sport, will be an eye-opener.

Figures 1.1a, 1.1b, 1.1c, and 1.1d illustrate this quite nicely for the 1,500-meter swim, 40-km bike time trial, marathon run,[2] and Ironman World Triathlon Championship in Kona, Hawaii.[3] Here you can see both world (swim, run, and Ironman) and U.S. national (bike) records by age group and gender. On the left side of each chart (the y-axis) are the record times; across the bottom (x-axis) are the age groups.

FIGURE 1.1A. **1500 m swim world records**

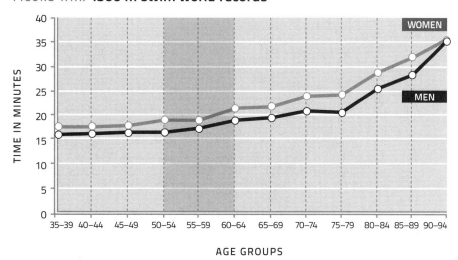

Source: Adapted from L. B. Ransdell, J. Vener, and J. Huberty, "Masters Athletes: An Analysis of Running, Swimming and Cycling Performance by Age and Gender," *Journal of Exercise Science and Fitness* 7 (2) (2009): S61–S73.

FIGURE 1.1B. **40 km U.S. cycling time trial records**

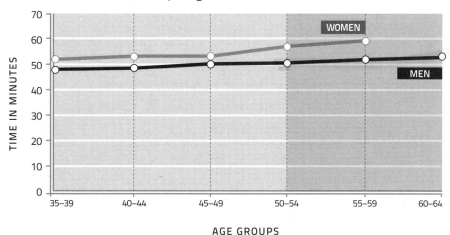

Source: Adapted from L. B. Ransdell, J. Vener, and J. Huberty, "Masters Athletes: An Analysis of Running, Swimming and Cycling Performance by Age and Gender," *Journal of Exercise Science and Fitness* 7 (2) (2009): S61–S73.

FIGURE 1.1C. **Marathon world records**

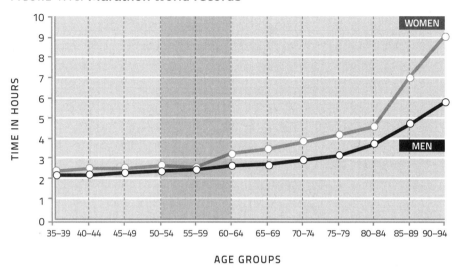

Source: Adapted from L. B. Ransdell, J. Vener, and J. Huberty, "Masters Athletes: An Analysis of Running, Swimming and Cycling Performance by Age and Gender," *Journal of Exercise Science and Fitness* 7 (2) (2009): S61–S73.

FIGURE 1.1D. **Ironman Triathlon World Championship records**

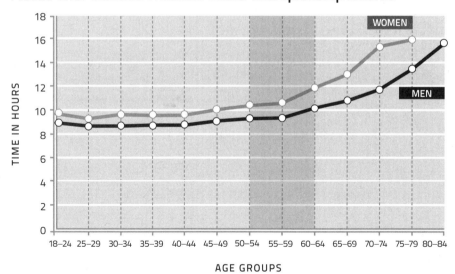

Source: Adapted from L. B. Ransdell, J. Vener, and J. Huberty, "Masters Athletes: An Analysis of Running, Swimming and Cycling Performance by Age and Gender," *Journal of Exercise Science and Fitness* 7 (2) (2009): S61–S73.

There are definite trends illustrated by these charts. It's obvious that even the very best age-group athletes slow down as they get older. We can also see that in the age groups from 50 to 59, there is a slightly more rapid decrease in performance (the times get slower, as indicated by rising chart lines). The decrease is most obvious in swimming and Ironman triathlon. We can also see that women's performances tend to decline faster than men's, especially in marathon running and Ironman triathlon. Swimming appears to have the least gender-related decline. By the record holders' mid- to late 70s and beyond, the performance slowdown increases markedly across all of the sports.

What's shown in these national- and world-record charts is generally in agreement with similar studies of elite age-group athletes in other competitive events. For example, researchers looked at the performances of senior Olympians (50 years and older) in the 2001 U.S. National Senior Olympic Games.[4] Both male and female performances declined by about 3 to 4 percent per year from age 50 to 85, but at a greater rate after age 75. Another study examined U.S. Masters Swimming Championship results from 1991 to 1995.[5] The researchers discovered a steady and linear decline in performance until about age 70, when performances started declining at a much faster rate. They also found that the declines were greater in women than in men.

Other researchers have observed similar rates of falling off in elite masters performances at national championships in swimming[6] and triathlon.[7] In the triathlon study, Ironman age-group performances declined at a greater rate than did those for the same age groups doing Olympic-distance (shorter) races. The study's authors suggested that the greater performance deterioration at the Ironman distance could be the result of an increased risk of injury and a more rapidly decreasing aerobic capacity because athletes who race at the longer distance train with greater durations and lower intensity than do short-course athletes. These are critical determiners of performance that we will return to many times in the coming chapters.

Of course, some of this dramatic change around age 70 may be due to societal effects. The leading edge of the baby-boom generation is just reaching its mid- to late 60s as of this writing. The running and fitness explosion began in the early 1970s, when the leading edge of that generation was in its late 20s. Many who were hooked then have been engaged in athletic performance ever since. These are the athletes who are now breaking age records in all sports.

The so-called silent generation, those born between 1929 and 1945, who came just before the baby boomers, didn't have the same exposure to sport and fitness. Growing up during the Great Depression, World War II, and the Cold War era had a lot to do with shaping that generation's values and lifestyles. Exercise, especially strenuous exercise, wasn't important. In fact, it was often frowned upon. People focused on career and family to the exclusion of sport and other "unnecessary" activities, and few became athletes. So those performance drop-offs in the charts for age groupers in their 70s and 80s may change dramatically in the coming years. We may soon see the records in all sports for the 70-year-old category significantly improve as the boomer generation "ages up." After all, that generation has been rewriting the record books for decades. Of course, this is pure conjecture on my part.

Given what these figures tell us, it seems that we can expect to measurably slow down at some point in our 50s, with a continuing decline that will bring the greatest negative rates of change in our 70s and beyond. Well, perhaps. All of this prediction and speculation on aging and performance is subject to change based on each individual's unique genetics and how serious that person is about the pursuit of athletic excellence.

Assuming you are currently facing what the best in the world have also experienced in terms of physiological decline, the key questions are: Why are these changes taking place? What can be done to slow them? We will look for answers to the first question in the next two chapters. We'll address the second question in Part II, where we will closely examine what can be done to slow the effects of age on performance. For now, though, let's look at what scientific research tells us about aging and athletic performance. The information is fascinating, and it also offers some important clues to the avenues we should pursue in order to maintain a high level of performance.

The Science of Aging

Since this chapter is devoted to understanding aging, and science offers the best way of doing so, we need to understand how such research is done. This may seem like needless detail, but it will help prevent us from chasing the wrong data for our decidedly non-normal purposes. So let's take a deeper look at where the numbers come from and how to use them.

Scientists face problems in their work, like everyone else. One of those problems is getting funding for their research—someone has to pay for all of that equipment and staff. Funding is generally scarce and comes primarily from four sources: government, business, foundations, and universities. Because money is hard to come by, researchers often seek ways to limit costs. When it comes to studying aging and physical performance, scientists often cut time and expense by conducting "cross-sectional" studies, which offer a quick look at the topic.

In cross-sectional research, the subjects chosen to be measured, poked, and prodded are assumed to represent most other people of their age and activity level. For example, if we were researching the effect of

age on a physiological indicator of performance such as body composition—that is, the effect of aging on how lean or how corpulent athletes
are—we might measure the body fat of a group of 20-something athletes
and also that of a group of athletes in their 60s. We may then assume
that the difference between the two groups is explained by age. The
problem with this assumption, of course, is that there could be other
factors affecting body composition such as how the subjects train (most
studies look only at training volume, not intensity) and even such seemingly insignificant details as income, lifestyle, marital status, time spent
watching television, diet, social mores, interests other than sport, and
lots more.

All of these things affect body composition in some small way. If we're
really good at science, we might be able to identify and control for some
of these factors, but we'll never be able to account for all of the possibilities. People are unique in many ways. We won't have enough time to even
learn what the differences are since contact time with the subjects is
quite limited. Cross-sectional studies are fairly easy to do, and since they
don't involve much time, they are also relatively inexpensive. As it happens, though, cross-sectional studies are not the gold standard when it
comes to aging.

The best research studies on aging are longitudinal. In a longitudinal
study of aging athletes, the same subjects are followed for a long time
with periodic tests and measurements. The researchers get to know the
subjects' training regimens, lifestyles, diets, daily activity levels, and
more. As you can imagine, much more meaningful conclusions can be
drawn about the effects of aging on body composition, or any other
physiological factor we want to understand, through a long-term study.
The longer the better. But we had better be willing to spend a lot of
money and time—years, perhaps decades. Our study may not be pub-

lished for 10 or 20 years. That's a big chunk of our lives devoted to gathering a limited amount of data. But for our purpose in understanding aging, these are the studies we want to know more about due to their considerable insights.

To understand where we are heading with all of this research stuff, we also need a basic understanding of exercise science. Regardless of age, there are only three things you can modify in a workout— *frequency, duration,* and *intensity.* Here are the most critical points for each.

Frequency. Exercise science research over the past several decades has shown that workouts must occur frequently in order to produce optimal results.[8] You must work out often to experience positive changes in performance. Big gaps in training cause losses in fitness that are very difficult to overcome.

Duration. Just as for young athletes, workouts for senior athletes must be sufficiently long to stimulate physiological changes.[9] If your sessions are too brief for the event you are training for, you can expect a lackluster performance due to poor aerobic endurance.

Intensity. We will study intensity (how hard the workout is) extensively throughout the remaining chapters, as it is a key tool for aging athletes.

There's one additional marker, volume, that you have almost certainly used in your training plans. Volume is simply the combination of frequency and duration—workout length times repetition over a fixed period. For example, if you did six 2-hour workouts in a week, your volume for that week would be 12 hours.

Now, let's apply all of this science to real-world athletes.

Research on Aging

For longitudinal studies of older athletes, we obviously have to step way back in time.

Bruce Dill and his colleagues at the Harvard University Fatigue Laboratory were among the first to apply the science of physiology to exercise. They conducted what was probably the original longitudinal study of aging in athletes, and it is also one of the best because of how long the athletes were followed—more than 20 years, starting in 1936.[10] In the first year of the study, 16 high-performance distance runners were tested for several factors including VO_2max. VO_2max, also known as aerobic capacity, is a marker of fitness that has to do with how much oxygen your body is capable of using when producing high levels of power. You'll come to understand VO_2max as an especially important determiner of performance with aging, and we'll return to it often in the following chapters.

Among Dill's 16 high-caliber subjects was a notable Indiana University runner by the name of Don Lash. At the time, Lash held the world record for the 2-mile distance (8:58) and had set the U.S. mark for the 10,000 meters (31:06).[11] Dill expected quite an extraordinary VO_2max for an athlete of this quality, and he wasn't disappointed. Lash tested at an exceptionally high 81.4 ml/kg/min (I'll explain all of this physiology mumbo jumbo in a later chapter; for now, take my word for it that this is an impressive figure). In those days, after graduation, very few former college runners continued to train. There were more pressing challenges during the Great Depression. Lash was an exception. He continued to run after leaving college, albeit with decreasing intensity and volume. By age 49, he was running about 45 minutes a day. (That, by the way, was not considered a short duration for a running workout in those days. Even in 1954, when Roger Bannister broke the 4-minute "barrier" for the mile, he was running about 45 minutes a day and typically only 5 days a week.

Before the 1970s, it was common for runners to avoid training on the weekends. My, how things have changed.)

Dill retested Lash at age 49. Some 25 years after the first test in the Harvard lab, Lash's VO_2max had dropped from 81.4 to 54.4—a decrease of 27 percent. At roughly 1 percent per year, that's really not too bad. Very few people around age 50 have such a high level of fitness. The other 15 former college runners who had initially been tested along with Lash back in 1936 had all stopped running by the follow-up test two and a half decades later. As might be expected, with little activity their loss was greater—about 43 percent, on average. That's just under 2 percent per year. In fact, in terms of VO_2max, they were no different than their sedentary peers who had never run.

Is there a take-home message from Dill's research on aging as it relates to Don Lash and the other subjects? One lesson is that having been in good physical condition earlier in life doesn't guarantee that you will continue to be fit later in life. This is just another case of an oft-quoted concept I'm sure you've come to understand: Use it or lose it. We'll pursue this particular lesson later on.

Lash's story may also be telling us something about the two major components of training—volume and intensity. Both the length of his workouts and how vigorous they were decreased over the years, but the intensity change was the greater of the two. As a consequence of a somewhat reduced training load, he lost a chunk of his fitness. Or would that have happened anyway just due to aging? Was the loss attributable to his genes or his reduced training? Let's pursue that question through another longitudinal study. This time we don't have to go quite so far back.

Another giant in the field of research on exercise, who was born in the same year Don Lash was being tested in Bruce Dill's Harvard lab, was Michael Pollock (he died in 1998). As director of research at the Institute for Aerobics Research in Dallas, Texas, he led one of the other classic longitudinal studies on aging.[12]

In the 1970s, 24 masters track runners, ages 42 to 59, were evaluated in the Texas lab by Dr. Pollock for VO_2max and body composition. Ten years later, they were retested. All of the subjects had continued to run in the intervening 10 years, but only 11 of them were still racing competitively. The members of this competitive group continued to run at a pace within about 30 seconds per mile of their pace 10 years prior. The other 13 had quit racing and reduced their exercise intensity accordingly. They were running about 90 seconds slower per mile than their earlier pace. Essentially, they did what many of us do as we get north of 50—we gravitate to long, slow distance (LSD) exercise. Both groups were still running at the same volume, within about 4 miles per week of where they'd been when first tested.

So what did Dr. Pollock find? The competitive, high-intensity group experienced an insignificant 1.6 percent drop in VO_2max, from 54.2 to 53.3 ml/kg/min. That's remarkable for a 10-year period. Unfortunately, the LSD group saw its VO_2max plummet from 52.5 to 45.9—more than 12 percent in 10 years. That's a rate of decline similar to Lash's, who had also taken up LSD training.

Pollock didn't stop there, however. He let another 10 years go by and then retested 21 of the original 24 athletes, who were now in their 60s and 70s.[13] Nine of them still trained with high intensity, 10 worked out with LSD at a moderate intensity, and the remaining 2 had greatly reduced both their training volume and intensity.

Things changed a bit now. The 9 competitive runners had lost 15 percent of their VO_2max over the intervening 10 years, dropping from 53 to 45—1.5 percent per year. Not bad.

And the 10 who continued to train at a moderate intensity? They saw a drop of 14 percent. Now, wait a second—how could they have lost less fitness than the more serious runners? The answer lies in where their previous levels had been. Having started at a lower number 10 years previously, they had less to lose, and their decline continued at about the same rate per year. So even though their percentage of decline was a bit smaller, their overall fitness was considerably lower.

And the two slow, low-volume joggers? They lost, on average, a whopping 34 percent of their VO_2max. That's 3.4 percent per year.

From this study, we may draw the conclusion that both training volume and intensity are important to the maintenance of fitness as we age, but intensity is more important. If true, this conclusion holds significant implications for how you should train: Maintain your weekly volume (hours, miles, or kilometers) if possible, but place a great emphasis on how hard your workouts are. Is this realistic as you age? Yes, it is, as we'll see in a moment.

But first, let's look a bit more closely at the intensity issue. So far, the conclusion that intensity should be maintained and is more important than volume when it comes to aging is based on only a few subjects in two studies. Since this is such a critical point, let's briefly look at the results of some additional longitudinal research.

Since the release of Pollock's original work, there have been several other longitudinal studies of aging endurance athletes. Four of the more recent ones are notable because they looked at changes in VO_2max relative to training volume and intensity.[14] They all got results similar to both Dill's and Pollock's studies. Essentially, what they found is that reducing the intensity of training as one gets older is a sure way to experience a drop in VO_2max. As you'll see later, VO_2max is one of your keys to high performance as an aging athlete. Continuing to train with high intensity results in roughly half as much decline as training with long, slow distance only.

The takeaway: Although volume is important, workout intensity is vital. In other words, you're better off reducing the volume of your training than reducing its intensity. Many aging athletes do just the opposite—a mistake that the programs in this book will help you avoid.

One of the more recent studies found an interesting twist that is thought-provoking.[15] The least-vigorous group of athletes in this study, those who did only LSD, saw their VO_2max drop 4.6 percent per year. That's huge. But here's the kicker: These LSD folks lost fitness at three times the annual rate of the sedentary, nonexercising subjects in the same study. This particular result has been confirmed by another, similar study.[16] Does that mean it's better to be sedentary?

The answer is *no*. The lesson is that if you greatly reduce your training, especially its intensity, your fitness will decline faster per year than will that of your nonexercising neighbors. That's because you are starting from a much higher number. In other words, since they are currently closer to the lowest number possible, they don't have much room left to fall. You, on the other hand, currently have a relatively high level of fitness; there's a great deal to lose by becoming sedentary or even just cutting back on intensity. Again: Use it or lose it.

Up to this point, we've seen an indirect emphasis on intensity based on a few longitudinal studies. In each of these studies, the conclusion that intensity is important wasn't determined until all of the training and lifestyle data on the subjects were examined several years later. That is, none of those studies started out intending to find the effect of intensity on performance. They were seeking to discover *what*, not *why*. They were observational studies that began with a question about what happens to athletes as they get older and in the process discovered why it happens.

If we want to examine only the effect of intensity on aging athletes, we need to look at a different type of study, one that controls for frequency and duration so that intensity is the only variable remaining. Of course it still needs to be longitudinal—the longer the better.

A study of this type is difficult to do because the scientists must ask serious athletes to change how they train for long periods of time. Athletes, regardless of age, tend to resist such manipulations. But it's been done: Another classic study examines the effect of workout intensity on fitness.[17] The main author, Professor Douglas Seals of the University of Colorado, has devoted his career to studying the benefits of aerobic exercise on older people. Who better to ask?

In Seals's study, seven men and four women (the first time any of the research we've looked at included women subjects), ranging in age from 61 to 67, trained for one year under the guidance of the scientists. For six months they trained with low intensity; for the other six months, with high intensity. The frequency (how often) and duration (how long) of their workouts remained the same, regardless of intensity. Along with several other markers of fitness, the VO_2max of each athlete was measured at the start and end of each six-month period.

The results? After the low-intensity period of training, VO_2max rose 12 percent. Very good. But after the high-intensity period, it rose 18 percent. Even better.

The takeaway from the Seals study: All exercise is good, but vigorous, high-intensity exercise produces greater benefits in aerobic fitness.

So what do we know now? Is there a solid message from all of this aging research? In fact, it should be quite clear: Intensity is the key to maintaining performance with aging.

Trainability and Aging

This emphasis on intensity may raise questions in your mind: Can older athletes adapt to the stresses of training as well as young athletes can? Are they able to physically cope with high-intensity workouts?

It appears that they can, at least in the short term. An occasional high-intensity workout is possible for nearly any senior athlete. The challenge we face is recovering from such workouts and repeating them day after day, week after week. And the task becomes more difficult as we age. Age is probably the greatest determiner of how frequently we can repeat such workouts, because recovery slows as the birthday candles pile onto the cake. We will examine all of these issues in upcoming chapters, along with how to best organize your training to optimize the adaptive process relative to your capacity for high-intensity workouts while avoiding the common pitfalls—injury, burnout, excessive fatigue, and overtraining.

For now, let me pass along another important discovery: The benefits of vigorous training aren't just the domain of the youngest of the senior athletes. Not only those in their 50s and 60s but also people in their 70s and 80s have been shown to benefit from strenuous training.[18] There may well be some good excuses for not training intensely, but age isn't one of them. More on that later.

The Aging Myth

In our society, and even among athletes, there is a common belief that growing old is fraught with devastating and unavoidable changes that are out of our control. The best you can hope for is to keep them at bay as long as possible by taking handfuls of pills every day. There is a parallel belief that you must not do anything vigorous. Protect your fragile bones. Stop strenuous exercising. Don't get your heart rate too high. Slow down. Take up gardening or bird watching. Act your age.

I suspect you are not buying into all of this. You've undoubtedly learned that the best antidote for the ravages of age is exercise. If for no other reason, you can see this in the differences between you and your normal neighbors. While you may be about the same chronological age, you are physiologically much younger than they are. Exercise, especially vigorous exercise, is powerful medicine. How powerful is it? That's where we're headed next.

THE AGELESS ATHLETE

Better to wear out than to rust out.

—JACK LALANNE

Before going any further, let's review two of the central themes of Chapter 1. A few points made there are critical to your purpose in reading this book. First, exercise keeps you healthy and much younger than what is normal for our society. Moreover, that exercise does not have to be highly intense to foster excellent health and allow you to lead a robust life as you get older. The subjects in the studies described in Chapter 1 who trained primarily with long, slow distance were much more fit and healthy than those who didn't. Exercise, regardless of intensity, is powerful medicine when it comes to health.

Second, and equally important *for athletes*: High-intensity exercise has a purpose beyond health. It improves endurance performance. You will race faster when you include intensity in your training.

If your reason for exercising is to live a long life filled with vibrant family activity and fun for many years to come, and you don't really care about how fast you are, then vigorous and frequent exercise of any type, including long, slow distance, is the way to go. In this chapter, we will examine why such a lifestyle works its magic—for, regardless of training intensity, health is the foundation on which fitness is built. If you aren't healthy, then high performance, regardless of how you may train, is unattainable. In Chapter 3, we'll start pulling all of these loose ends together and show you how to train for performance. For now, let's take a closer look at exercise and its amazing effect on how you age.

Exercise as Medicine

Scientists who study aging would love to know what makes you tick.[1] Your unusual lifestyle as an older, active athlete holds the secrets to health and longevity. For example, obesity among those over the age of 60 is rapidly increasing, yet you undoubtedly eat more and still weigh less than your nonexercising age peers. Even better, your risk of coronary artery disease is probably much lower than that of normal old folks. Your chance of contracting type 2 diabetes, which is associated with the risk factors of eating too much of the wrong foods and not exercising enough—the black plague of the 21st century—is also quite low. Only 13 percent of people beyond age 65 exercise vigorously three or more days a week.[2] And yet you feel guilty when you take a day off.

Why do you do it? What motivates you? Why do you exercise regularly when you could much more easily sit comfortably in a rocking chair? Why do you concern yourself with the foods you eat and voluntarily limit your portions? Scientists would like to capture whatever you have so it could be given to others—probably as a pill, since that is how we seem to solve all health problems in our society. They've certainly been searching for the answers. What they've found from interviews of older athletes is that they exercise for many reasons, such as the psychological challenge of competition, a desire to measure themselves against others, feelings of accomplishment, the health benefits of exercise, and social interaction with like-minded people.[3]

It would be hard to put these motivators into a pill. You either have them or you don't. Most don't. That's why you aren't normal. So what does makes you tick?

So far, about all science knows about exercise and aging is that there seems to be an inverse relationship between older people's volume of exercise and their risk of premature death, regardless of the cause.[4] In other words, the more you exercise, the less likely you are to die early. Some of this research has even come up with specific numbers.[5] If you burn about 1,000 "extra" calories (technically, these would be kilocalories, but to avoid confusion we will use the more common term in this book) per week in exercise, the risk of early death is reduced by more than 20 percent. A thousand calories isn't much; you burn those in roughly two to three hours of exercise in a week. Yet you probably do that and much more. That's good. The more calories you expend, the lower your risk.[6]

Of course, there is more to life than just how long you live. Quality is at least as important as quantity. Living a long time in loneliness and boredom, with little in the way of activity except for occasional exercise, is not what any of us want. Quality of life means not only participation in sport as an athlete but also simply being an energetic and a dynamic person in all aspects of life. Growing old in front of a television is not what endurance athletes generally think of as fun.

The longitudinal studies you read about in Chapter 1 were done in order to understand all of this. The scientists wanted to know what happens to athletes as they age, not only in terms of performance but also in regard to the many common measures of health such as body composition, heart function, and muscular strength. Along the way they also discovered the secrets to high performance with aging.

I should point out that there are a few studies suggesting that extreme exercise, such as frequent marathons or Ironman triathlons done at a relatively high intensity, could put unnatural stresses on your heart and may actually shorten your life compared with the life expectancy of athletes who do fewer and shorter events.[7] There are lingering questions, however, about the accuracy of these studies, particularly in regard to the self-selected research subjects.[8] Did they volunteer because they had a sense that they were at high risk for heart disease? If so, then we may be seeing biased results.

What we can say, though, is that the rest and recovery you give your body are critical. As with nearly everything in life, moderation appears to be the key. For athletes, this means being thoughtful and realistic about the frequency of your most challenging workouts and races. You will see this issue addressed in later chapters, where we explore how to organize your training to get optimal benefits without undue stress. In the meantime, please bear in mind that overexercising is certainly possible. Attempting frequent high-intensity and long-duration workouts may actually compromise your health and your life expectancy. If you have doubts about your heart health, then it's probably wise to talk with your doctor about the need for testing.

Of Mice and Men

As we've seen so far, what we thought we knew about normal aging isn't really normal for humans at all. Senior athletes provide proof of that every time they race. Many continue to perform better than much younger athletes. These older athletes can do it because they have the right genes, and they continue to push their physical and mental limits. They're unwilling to accept a number as a reason that they can't do it. While aging does inevitably take a toll on the performance of aging athletes, it's small compared with the loss of functional performance that normal, inactive people experience due to disuse. Most people "rust out" due to inactivity rather than "wear out" from being overly active.

Strenuous exercise is a key to not only the quality of life but also its quantity—how long we live. This is difficult for science to verify, as university ethics committees charged with approving study protocols aren't big on manipulating human subjects' lifestyles to see who lives longer. That leaves us with animal studies on the effects of exercise on health and longevity. Mice are commonly used in such research because they have fairly short lifespans; studying the effects of aging in mice can be done rather quickly.

One such aging-and-exercise study using mice was done at McMaster University in Hamilton, Ontario, Canada, a few years ago.[9] Mice that were bred to age rapidly were divided into two groups. One group was sedentary. The other group ran on treadmills three times per week for 45 minutes, each time at a brisk pace that was the equivalent of a 50- to 55-minute 10-km run for humans. By 8 months, which is roughly age 60 for humans, the sedentary mice were frail, gray, and dying.

Figure 2.1 shows two of the subject mice. On the left is an exerciser. On the right is a sedentary mouse of the same age (30 weeks). There's a visible difference in their physiological ages.

All of the sedentary mice were dead by 12 months of age. But at that same age, the exercisers were still looking and acting young. Not one had died.

Now we know that exercise produces mice that look young and live a long time. But what about humans?

FIGURE 2.1. **Exercising and nonexercising mice in late life**

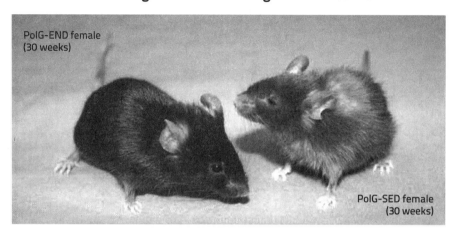

PolG-END female
(30 weeks)

PolG-SED female
(30 weeks)

Source: A. Safdar, J. Bourgeois, D. I. Ogburn, J. P. Little, B. P. Hettinga, M. Akhtar, J. E. Thompson, S. Melov, N. J. Mocellin, G. C. Kujoth, T. A. Prolla, and M. A. Tarnopolsky, "Endurance Exercise Rescues Progeroid Aging and Induces Systemic Mitochondrial Rejuvenation in mtDNA Mutator Mice," *Proceedings of the National Academy of Sciences USA* 108 (10) (2011). Used with permission.

Telomeres

In addition to candles on a birthday cake, there are many ways to measure how old someone is. Take telomeres, for example. Telomeres are the caps on the ends of your DNA strands. Every time a cell in your body divides to produce a new cell, its telomeres get slightly shorter. When the telomeres reach a minimum length, they can no longer continue to shorten. At that point, the cell can no longer divide, which marks the beginning of the end—senescence.

Since telomeres are decent predictors of longevity, scientists use them as markers of cell age and therefore physiological age, which may vary greatly from biological age. The longer a cell's telomeres, the younger the cell is, regardless of the number of years it's been on the planet.

The length of telomeres is also closely related to VO_2max and therefore endurance performance. Longer is better both for longevity and for performance. So how long are your telomeres? And can you slow the shortening of your telomeres with exercise?

A few years ago scientists at the University of Colorado in Boulder measured the telomeres of young (age 18 to 32) and old (age 55 to 72) subjects.[10] Each age group was divided into two subgroups—sedentary and endurance-trained—creating four groups in all. When the telomeres of old, sedentary subjects were compared with those of the young, sedentary subjects, the oldsters' were 16 percent shorter. They really were "old." The telomeres of the old, endurance-trained subjects, however, were only 7 percent shorter than those of the endurance-trained youngsters. That is to say, old athletes had telomeres that were 13 percent longer than those of their sedentary peers. Telomere length was directly related to activity level. Even though science can't explain why, exercise slows aging by keeping your telomeres young. And where your telomeres go, so go you. Once again we see that exercise is, indeed, powerful medicine.

We also know from the longitudinal studies of athletes in Chapter 1 that the more intensely you train, the greater your VO_2max. And that means improved endurance performance. Telomeres, training intensity, VO_2max, and performance are all related in some way. Could it be that the more aerobically fit you are, the longer you live? That question hasn't been definitively answered by scientists yet. But we're getting closer, as you'll see.[11]

Theories of Aging

Interestingly, not all of Earth's creatures are afflicted by shortening telomeres. Take the planarian flatworm, for example. This tiny worm's telomeres seem to have an unlimited ability to regenerate and preserve length.[12] Planaria can restore any part of the body—from brain to digestive system—and maintain life indefinitely. They appear to be ageless, even immortal. As you may imagine, some scientists who study aging are taking a very close look at the flatworm.

The closest we humans come to having cells that last indefinitely happens to be cancer. Unfortunately, cancer cells are close to being immortal because their telomeres somehow maintain their length as they divide, thus avoiding senescence. That's what makes cancer such a dreadful disease.

How is it that some human cells can divide without shortening their telomeres? Scientists are trying to answer that question. Others are looking at how a cancer cell's telomeres can be prevented from maintaining their length with regeneration in order to gain control of the disease once it appears.[13] Hastening the shortening of cancer telomeres could kill off the cells. But aside from cancer treatment and from a strictly aging point of view, messing around with human telomeres in order to extend life may actually increase our risk of contracting cancer.[14] There's a lot yet to be learned about telomeres.

What we know for certain is that the older your body's cells become, the fewer years you have left. From what we've learned from mice and from human athletes, it's apparent that exercise plays a major role in longevity. This is at the heart of a pressing matter for our society: the financial cost of maintaining an aging population. Since the 1960s, when aging became a hot topic in the United States due to the overall population increase from the baby-boom generation coupled with the introduction of Medicare and Medicaid, scientists have been trying to understand why we age. Their curiosity has been motivated by an interest not only in extending human life but also in controlling government expenditures, such as medical costs and Social Security, in support of longer-living citizens. The U.S. Bureau of Labor Statistics estimates that by the year 2020, one-quarter of working Americans will be over the age of 55 and approaching retirement.[15] How will the government support so many retirees? Understanding aging, especially the health of older people, is critical to finding solutions.

The starting point for understanding anything in science is having a theory—in this case, a theory about what causes aging. Is telomere shortening a cause or merely a result of the aging process? If it's a result, which many scientists believe, what is the root cause? The following is a brief look at a few of the more popular theories from the past 50 years of what causes aging.

Heartbeat Theory

Some have speculated that all creatures have a certain number of heartbeats built in at conception, and when these heartbeats are used up, life ends. This rather simplistic theory came from observing animals with rapid heart rates and short life spans, such as rabbits and mice, and animals with slow heart rates that live a long time, such as elephants and whales. It's been noted that endurance athletes have very slow resting heart rates compared with nonathletes and also live longer.[16]

Wear-and-Tear Theory

This theory is based on the premise that the body is like a machine. Just as machines wear out with use, so does the human body. As you use your body's systems, such as your heart and lungs, over your lifetime, the systems develop signs of wear and tear at the molecular level and eventually are forced to stop functioning.[17] The excessive wear may also result from environmental factors such as solar radiation, air pollution, toxins in food, and exposure to X-rays.

Free-Radical Theory

This theory is a bit more complex version of the previous one, but you are probably familiar with it because it's been the most widely accepted theory of the reasons behind aging and the occurrence of disease for most of our adult lives.

As you breathe and metabolize food, your body creates by-products called "metabolites." Metabolites may be electrically neutral, or they may be positively or negatively charged by releasing or gaining an electron. The newly charged molecules are known as "free radicals." Free radicals want to return to a neutral-charge state, so they seek out other cells in the body in an attempt to gain or lose electrons. This process cascades through the body, creating more free radicals and further damaging other cells. It also weakens the cells, making them more prone to disease and speeding up the aging process. To offset this cascading effect, proponents of this theory place an emphasis on consuming free-radical-attaching antioxidants, either as food or as supplements.

This theory was introduced in 1956, became a popular explanation of the aging process by the 1980s,[18] and soon created an entire industry dedicated to producing antioxidant supplements such as beta-carotene, vitamin A, vitamin C (ascorbic acid), vitamin E, and selenium. Today, however, the free-radical theory appears to be in the early stages of demise. For example, scientists studying worms and mice have found that these critters live longer when certain free radicals are introduced into their bodies.[19] That's raised some eyebrows. Furthermore, recent research looking at several diseases once thought to be a result of free radicals suggests that antioxidant supplements are generally ineffective and may actually do more harm than good, especially if taken in excess.[20] The upshot? It's probably unwise to bombard your body with supplements. Instead, maintain a balanced diet and a balanced approach to your daily exercise and training routine, and you'll almost certainly come out ahead.

DNA Damage Theory

The DNA damage theory takes us back to the DNA strands where we found the telomeres earlier. As cells divide, naturally occurring changes in their DNA structure take place. These changes are known to happen as often as 7,000 times per hour in the cells of a mouse.[21] This could be due to a microscopic tear in one of the two twisted DNA strands or their cross-links or possibly to a residue buildup. The affected cell may be unable to replicate, which is necessary for the individual's health and longevity, or the cell may even die as a result.[22] Animals, including humans, have evolved to continuously repair these little breakdowns, but they aren't 100 percent successful. Some malfunctions are missed and go unrepaired. The supporters of this theory propose that these small, unmended damages accumulate over time, resulting in significant genomic changes and thus aging.

Programmed Theory

This theory proposes that death, and therefore aging, is built into all organisms by evolution. That is, if life is uninterrupted by environmental factors or disease, then every organism, including humans, will live for a certain number of years that falls within a narrow range. For example, we know that a worker bee lives about 1 year and a mouse about 4 years. An elephant's life span is roughly 80 years. The Galápagos land tortoise, currently considered the longest-living animal on the planet, trundles around for about 190 years. According to the World Health Organization, humans have a life expectancy, on average, of about 68 years, although life span varies by gender and location.[23] Females tend to live longer than males by roughly 5 years. The country with the highest age at death is Japan: 83 years on average. With life span seemingly more or less set, say the proponents of the programmed theory, the best we can hope for is to limit the external forces that shorten life. Lack of exercise is certainly a life-span shortener, so from that perspective, the programmed theory makes a certain amount of sense.

• • •

We've just touched the surface when it comes to theories of aging. There are many more, but the bottom line is that science doesn't yet know what causes aging and therefore death. It could be that none of these theories completely explain senescence, and new theories are likely to surface as scientists learn more about aging by studying the baby-boom generation. It could also be that aging involves several explanations.

Although we may not yet know what exactly causes us to become old, has science found any surefire method to slow the process of aging? Let's look for an answer.

Slower Aging

A handful of years ago, scientists at the Mayo Clinic in Rochester, Minnesota, came up with a novel way to reverse aging.[24] As you might suspect, the study was done using elderly mice, not baby boomers. The researchers gave the mice a drug that caused their senescent cells to self-destruct. These are the cells with telomeres that can no longer shorten, thus indicating that the cell is fully aged, damaged, or dysfunctional and possibly close to death. Such cells seem to have a negative effect on neighboring cells, causing them to age faster, too. The cells that were treated were in the eyes, muscles, and fat tissues. And something unusual happened. The late-life mice seemed to drink from the fountain of youth. They no longer developed cataracts in their eyes; their muscle tissues stopped wasting away; and the fat layers just below their skin no longer thinned out, which is what causes wrinkling in humans. And the mice were able to run much longer on a mouse treadmill. They were young again.

It's doubtful that removing senescent cells will ever become a common "therapy" for aging humans in our lifetimes. But this research produces hope that aging might someday be slowed down, if not completely reversed, by taking a pill.

Of course you, as an athlete, have already found the fountain of youth. You drink from it daily. The most powerful antiaging "pill" available to humans is exercise.

> YOU, AS AN ATHLETE, have already found the fountain of youth. You drink from it daily.

We know for certain that exercise slows if not reverses the aging process. That's essentially what we saw happening with the runners in the longitudinal studies we looked at in Chapter 1. Functional performance, whether it involves getting out of a chair unassisted or running a 10K race, is one of the best indicators of how old you really are. Exercise helps to keep your telomeres from shortening as fast as they do for your normal neighbors. Let's take a look at how that happens.

Stem Cells

The exact process that causes cells to degrade with aging is not completely understood, but inflammation, traumatic injury, and disease can certainly play a role in their demise. Disuse is another common cause and perhaps the most prevalent in Western society. How could disuse degrade a cell? The answer seemingly lies in stem cells, microscopic organelles that spring into action to start repair when a muscle cell is damaged in some way.

The muscles of young people are replete with stem cells. A normal process of aging is for these stem cells to die off, resulting in sarcopenia—muscle wasting. The muscles are no longer maintained. Research at Tel Aviv University has shown, however, that exercise is the key to keeping stem cells alive and functioning.[25]

In the Tel Aviv study, a group of formerly sedentary rats of varying ages ran on a treadmill for 20 minutes daily for 13 weeks. Another pack of rats was the control group. The control group was allowed to remain sedentary—that is, those rats' muscles were mainly not used. As you might expect from everything you've read so far, the exercisers increased their number of stem muscle cells, with the total increase dependent on age—but not in the way you would expect. The younger rat runners saw an increase of 20 to 35 percent in their stem repair cells. The older rats, however, experienced an even greater proliferation—a 33 to 47 percent increase. That's right: The percentage increase in stem muscle cells was greater in the older subjects than in the younger ones. On the other hand, the nonexercising rats lost stem cells by lying around, eating and sleeping as they aged.

By now you may be thinking that this chapter contains a lot of good news for rodents—but people are different. You're right; they are in some small ways. But research on humans employing both endurance and muscular strength training has shown that such exercise generates a cascade of naturally made molecules in the tissues surrounding the exercised muscles, resulting in an increase in stem-cell activity.[26] So it's not just rat and mouse muscles that benefit from exercise. Furthermore, such research on humans has demonstrated that highly intense exercise produces a greater benefit in this regard than just slogging along at a low intensity.[27] That finding includes oldsters as well as youngsters.[28]

Where have we seen the benefits of high-intensity exercise before? Remember the longitudinal studies of runners? The more intensely they exercised, the more slowly their fitness declined. Could this be because their stem cells were renewing muscles? That's certainly possible. But even without ironclad proof of the involvement of stem cells, the bottom line is more evidence that exercise improves muscle health and keeps you younger than your years. It slows how rapidly you age.

ANDREW
PRUITT,
EdD

Sports Equipment and Aging

As a soon-to-be 64-year-old, I definitely fall into the category of a senior endurance athlete. My sports of choice are cycling and classic Nordic skiing. As a sports medicine provider for over 40 years, I have watched not only myself but also hundreds of patients age. I actually have patients whom I have known and cared for over the entire span of my practice. Some were college kids who are now in their late 50s, and some were adults before they crossed my table who are now as old as 80-plus. I have made several observations as we have all aged together.

The most poignant is that at some point we can no longer outrun our gene pool! In our youth and even middle age we can eat right, exercise, use sunscreen, and look and feel marvelous "for our age." But there comes a time when we suddenly begin to look like our parents or grandparents. The disease and aging processes that have some genetic, historical, or environmental influence catch up with us. I have observed this in patients, friends, and now myself.

My parents were both heavy smokers, so until the age of 17 I lived with heavy secondhand smoke. As a youngster I was more of a sprinter and an explosive athlete. The loss of maximum pulmonary function didn't really become an issue until my mid-30s, when I was a masters bike racer. Now, as a senior endurance athlete, I would love to have back those smoke-filled years—without the smoke. A larger tidal lung volume would make the long Colorado canyon climbs a bit more comfortable for me, if not faster. My family also had a tendency to be a little generous around the middle (isolated middle-age belly fat). I was able to avoid it with exercise and diet until about age 55, at which point the old gene pool came calling, regardless of my righteous routine.

Cardiopulmonary disease, body composition, and biomechanics are all impossible to fully avoid. Just like driving a car that is a little out of »

Continued

alignment: You are going to drive it, maybe even drive it hard, and all of a sudden the tires (knees) are unevenly worn. Joints and tendons are the same. It is as if they have a wear bar, and beyond a certain level of wear, they begin to hurt. Patients say, "I have been running for 20 years, and they never hurt me before. What did I do wrong?" The answer is nothing—you just lived life. This is not the place to discuss what we can do at that point, but I am not giving up, and I don't suggest you do so, either. But we may have to change things as we age.

A couple of years ago, I was marveling at my nearly 60-year-old colleague Ned Overend's perpetual fitness. I asked him how he did it. He said, "I do exactly what I have always done; it just takes me longer to get it done." What he was saying is that a 4-week training block now takes him 6 to 8 weeks to accomplish due to the added recovery time. This recovery takes many forms. This surely happened to me, but before I thought about it correctly, I was finding myself overreached, over-trained, or just plain exhausted from not letting myself recover. I surely was not giving work, travel, and stress appropriate consideration, either. Thanks for the tip, Ned!

Equipment choices are a crucial part of maintaining an athletic lifestyle as we age. My bike position is a bit more relaxed than it was in »

Okinawans

Could there be ways to slow the process of aging besides exercise? In interviewing people who have lived to be 100, journalists have found all sorts of reasons given by the superseniors for their longevity. Some will swear by a cigar a day, while others will say they never touched tobacco. Some used marijuana, some didn't; some drank plenty of alcohol, others abstained. Some ate meat, some ate lots of fat, some ate only vegetables. Some stayed active, some sat on the front porch. Although these inter-

my youthful racing days. Not that my bike looks like a beach cruiser—trust me, it is still a race position—but it reflects my aging back, hands, and shoulders. Tire choice and pressure are things we may rarely think about, but making the right choices there can significantly improve ride comfort. The aging prostate gland needs to have some consideration as well. Part of bike fit for the senior should consider reducing the pressure and vibration on your perineum. I suggest that the senior cyclist work with a good professional bike fitter and equipment consultant.

Running-shoe technology has also come a long way from the original waffle trainer on which I consulted many years ago. Senior runners should get their gear advice from a professional, not a teenager in a striped shirt at the mall or online.

I have found a young sports-medicine-trained internist for my personal doctor. I wanted a relatively young, well-trained physician who respected my athletic past and future and who encouraged and supported my continued sporting life. I still want to ride 5,000 miles and Nordic ski 400 to 600 kilometers per year. I don't tell my patients, "Well, if it hurts, don't do it," and I didn't want that for myself, either. I suggest that you find a similar medical practitioner for your senior athletic years!

views can be fun to read, they don't give us much useful guidance on how to live our lives.

A more accurate way to find what is associated with living a long time is to study the lifestyles of a large number of old people to see what they have in common other than good genetics. These other factors may not be quite as effective as exercise since, as we've seen, exercise is perhaps the most potent antiaging method available. But even one or two changes in the way we live may slow aging even more. Slowing the aging process also means staying healthier and more physically active for a longer time. Perhaps by examining the lifestyles of centenarians—people who have been around for 100 years or more—we can find one or two more of these relatively small fountains of youth. Of course, it could just be that we'll only find people who won the longevity lottery, those who had the right parents. However, there may be some common threads among those who live a long time—threads that may allow us to stay young at the cellular level with longer telomeres and an abundance of stem cells.

In fact, such studies have been done of the long-living residents on the island of Okinawa, a Japanese prefecture in the Pacific Ocean. Historically, Okinawans have lived a long time. In industrialized countries, it is common to find 10 to 20 people out of every 100,000 who live 100 years or more. In Okinawa, there are more than twice as many—40 to 50 centenarians per 100,000.[29] That's the most of any place on earth we know of.

Could this be solely a story about genetics? Or might lifestyle also play a role in Okinawan aging? That is, is it nature or nurture? The answer may surprise you.

For centuries, Okinawa's location as a tiny island in the Pacific midway between Japan and Taiwan protected its residents from outsiders and helped to maintain their ancestral lifestyle. World War II changed that. Okinawa was the only Japanese land on which there was fighting. In the spring of 1945, an American amphibious assault, the largest of the war in the Pacific, lasted 82 days. One-third of the island's population died in the fighting. As you can imagine, the Battle of Okinawa brought huge changes to the inhabitants' lifestyle. The most significant changes occurred after the establishment of an American military base in the aftermath of the war. The Okinawan lifestyle was "Westernized." The change was apparent in two areas—physical activity and diet.

Prior to the war, the Okinawan centenarians seemed to benefit not only from their genes, which were certainly impressive, but also from manual labor and lots of walking. Cars were rare before the U.S. occupation. The traditional Okinawan diet included pork, fresh fish, and lots of vegetables and was very low in sugar and other highly refined carbohydrates.[30] Compared with mainland Japanese, Okinawans ate little in the way of grains, including rice, but they ate more sweet potatoes.[31] In addition, ancient Okinawan customs included eating just enough to satisfy the appetite. Their cultural heritage was to eat until 80 percent full, known as *"hara hachi bu."* Eating foods that were low in sugar but rich in protein, healthy fats, and fiber made this "undereating" possible because those foods satisfy the appetite more quickly. Indeed, several research studies have demonstrated that caloric restriction seems to lengthen the lives of animals and may benefit human life expectancy as well.[32]

All of this began changing when the first McDonald's opened on the island in 1976.[33] Now fast-food restaurants are prolific and do a brisk business. Okinawans today eat like Americans—hamburgers, French fries, and soft drinks are common. They no longer walk from shop to shop for the necessities of life; shopping malls are abundant and easily accessible by car. Having at one time been the leanest of the Japanese citizens, the islanders, mostly the men, are now among the fattest, and their ranking as the longest-living people on the planet is rapidly falling. Centenarians are becoming as rare in Okinawa as in the United States.

In addition, scientists are finding that when young people move away from the island (another trend since the war) or otherwise adopt a Western diet and way of life, which are both much different from those of their ancestors, there is a decline in longevity.[34] Apparently, good genes can be trumped by a bad lifestyle.

So is it less physical activity, a dietary change to Western foods, or overeating that is causing the changes in health and longevity among genetically blessed Okinawans? Unfortunately, science has not been able to separate and appraise the changes to identify their individual contributions to the decline. Yet there are still lessons here. One I continue to drive home is that exercise, regardless of intensity, can lead to a long life. We know that. It's very well established. But the other message from the Okinawan experience, which we'll examine much more closely in Chapter 8, is that diet also has a lot to do with health and longevity. Gluttonous eating may also play a role. All of this is probably not a great revelation for you, but it sets the stage for where we are heading. Later we'll expand on these subjects as we examine how eating a diet that is age-appropriate may also benefit performance.

The Ageless Athlete

Is age just a number? Some senior athletes believe it is. They refuse to think of how old they are as an excuse. They insist that regardless of age, they expect to train and race at a high level. They exercise as if they are still young and energetic. Consequently, they are. Their athletic lifestyles also reflect this powerful and positive attitude. Eating is regarded as refueling and not as a recreational activity. Foods are chosen primarily for their healthful benefits rather than for gluttonous gratification. These athletes' training partners and friends are often much younger than they and just as dedicated to excellence. The ageless athlete's spouse may also be quite energetic and mentally youthful. They share a common goal: a long and healthy life filled with physical activity and high levels of achievement.

Yet even such a positive attitude coupled with an intense dedication to high performance doesn't stop the consequences of aging. Ever-shortening telomeres and disappearing stem cells still happen. Even the most resolute of athletes eventually experiences these age-related physical transformations. But somehow the negative effects are delayed and diminished. That's why science would love to know what makes older athletes tick. That information could change the world. But no one knows the answer—except you. You do it for many reasons, but chief among them is enjoyment. Training makes you feel as if you are a kid again. It's fun. Science will never come up with a pill that reproduces such an attitude. It's almost as if this is a part of our unique DNA.

For the serious senior athlete, fun includes high performance. Even if we're not competing with others, as many still are, we are at least competing with the greatest competitor of all—our younger selves. Beating personal performances from when we were younger brings a great sense of achievement. If it's been a while since you last accomplished that, what do you need to get back to such a high level of fitness? What's standing between you and great athletic performance? Understanding the challenge is the first step in conquering it. That's where we're going in Chapter 3.

3

OVER THE HILL

Never put an age limit on your dreams.

—DARA TORRES

At the 1984 Olympic Games in Los Angeles, Portugal's Carlos Alberto de Sousa Lopes won the gold medal in the marathon, setting a new Olympic record of 2:09:21. At age 38, he also set a record for being the oldest Olympic men's marathon winner in history, a record that still stands. The age record for the oldest women's Olympic marathon gold medalist also happens to be 38: Romanian runner Constantina Dita Tomescu ran 2:26:44 in Beijing in 2008. Those are records that are unlikely to be broken anytime soon, as the common age range of Olympic marathon winners is 25 to 35.

And it isn't just in the Olympics that we see such young winners. The top five women and men for the past decade at the World Marathon Majors—Chicago, London, New York, Berlin, and Boston—along with the Olympics and World Championships were 29 years old, plus or minus one year.[1]

The oldest track-and-field gold medalist at any Olympics was 42: Patrick McDonald, an American hammer thrower in the 1920 Games in Antwerp. The oldest athlete ever to medal in an Olympic endurance event was Germany's Sabine Spitz, who at age 40 took silver in women's cross-country mountain bike in 2012 in London. The oldest Olympic track champion in the 1,500-meter race was 31-year-old British runner Albert Hill in the 1920 Antwerp Games.

All of this means that you shouldn't expect to see many athletes who are 50 or older on the podium at the Olympics, World Championships, or other world-class endurance events. Even 40-somethings don't stand much of a chance. The gold medal usually goes to someone who is around 30.

If you've been training seriously in your sport for 10 years or more, you've undoubtedly experienced this loss firsthand. If you've been at it for just a handful of years, however, you may still be improving your race performances relative to young athletes, especially if you are in your 50s. It takes several years for endurance athletes to approach their potential once they start focused and consistent training, regardless of age.

Chapter 2 pointed out several of the genetic, cellular changes, from shortened telomeres to disappearing stem cells, that may eventually contribute to this loss of performance, along with a few unproven aging theories such as the currently popular free-radical hypothesis. These help us to explain the process of aging. We also learned in Chapter 2 that exercise plays an important role in slowing aging. Both the natural process of human aging, even if we don't fully understand it, and your chosen athletic lifestyle have produced and continue to produce who you are. These personal determiners—genetics and lifestyle—are often referred to as "nature" and "nurture." Obviously, both are important, but which is the more critical when it comes to how fast you lose (or gain) your capability for performance?

There is reason to believe that the major contributor to the performance decline in athletes as they get older is nurture, with nature playing a smaller role. This contradicts what our society has come to believe—that the vagaries of aging occur at a given rate, are inevitable, and are completely outside one's control. That line of thinking makes it easy to throw up your hands and surrender.

This doesn't mean that nature's effects are trivial. They are far from that. But a vigorous lifestyle—and especially strenuous activity, what I've been calling "high-intensity training"—has a powerful influence on physiology and has the power to keep old age and poor performance at bay. We saw this in the longitudinal studies in Chapter 1. Reduced training intensity resulted in marked changes in the performance-related physiology of the athlete subjects. The loss of a vigorous lifestyle may also explain, in part, the declining life span of Okinawans (alterations in their diet, another common nurture game-changer, may also be partly to blame).

> A VIGOROUS LIFESTYLE has the power to keep old age and poor performance at bay.

Some scientists who study sport and aging also see the balance tilted toward the nurture side because as we age, exercise behavior (nurture) appears to play a significant role in how our given genetic biology (nature) plays out.[2] The balance could be around 60–40 or even 70–30. In other words, 60 to 70 percent of our reduced performance might be explained by changes in training (and perhaps also by lifestyle in general), with the changes due to biological aging accounting for only 30 to 40 percent.

With that in mind, the chief question must be: What do we need to do to get the large nurture portion right so that we can stay fast after age 50? I firmly believe that the answer lies in high-intensity training, and that type of training will be our main focus going forward. There are additional ingredients, however, that I will address in Chapters 4 through 8. In each case, we'll be looking for more answers to our fundamental question of how we can stay fast and competitive throughout our athletic careers.

Before we get to that, however, we need to fully understand what we're up against. As a lifetime athlete, you know how important it is to have a smart race plan. If you know where the hills lie on the course, what obstacles to expect, and where you expect your competition to be especially strong, you can plan for a better race. And that's exactly how we should approach our goal.

The first question in our plan, therefore, is this: What physical performance changes are occurring as you become older? And I do mean *you*. Although the research indicates what senior athletes *generally* experience with aging, not all of those conclusions may apply to you. There is no reason to train for those things that may be true for aging athletes as a demographic group but don't seem to be limiting your performance. And our goal, clearly, is to optimize your athletic performance for years to come.

To get started on this question, perhaps the most important discovery you can make is to determine what is holding you back—your event-specific weakness (or, more commonly, weaknesses plural). I call these "limiters." Note that limiters are *event-specific* weaknesses. Not all weaknesses are limiters. For example, if you aren't good at very long endurance events but excel at short ones, endurance may be a weakness, but it's not necessarily a limiter. Having poor long-distance endurance is not holding you back if the events in which you compete are the 1-mile or 5K foot race rather than marathons and ultramarathons.

Many areas of your life could produce nurture limiters, such as the amount of time you have available to train, your diet, how much sleep you get, your speed of recovery, and much more. We'll get into some of these potential limiters in later chapters. But our focus now is on the big rocks—those few things in your training and lifestyle that may well be limiting your performance as an endurance athlete. Your purpose in this chapter is to determine your unique physiological limiters.

For nearly all senior athletes, the performance-related changes that are most common are what I call the "big three" aging limiters:

- Decreasing aerobic capacity
- Increasing body fat
- Shrinking muscles

We won't look for solutions for these yet. We will simply try to understand what seems to be going on with them and your body, if indeed all three apply to you. As you read what follows, you must decide whether the topic at hand seems to describe what is happening to *your* body. Is it *your* limiter? If so, pursue it. If not, be grateful and move on.

There are some additional possibilities besides these three that we will consider near the end of this chapter. By the time you have finished the chapter, you should be able to answer the critical question for the aging athlete: What is limiting my performance?

What Is Fitness?

Before we get into the details of what's happening to your body, and therefore your performance, let's take a look at what accounts for endurance performance in the first place—regardless of how old you are. When it comes to endurance sports, what is fitness?

Science tells us there are three physiological predictors of your endurance performance that hold true across the aging spectrum:

- Aerobic capacity
- Lactate threshold
- Economy

Some combination of your capabilities in each of these three areas helps to describe who you are as an athlete. Chances are that as a well-read and longtime student of endurance training, you are already familiar with these, at least in a general way. But let's summarize them to be sure we're on the same page, since so much of what follows is related.

Aerobic Capacity

Aerobic capacity is a measure of how much oxygen you use when exercising at a sustained, maximal workload. The more oxygen you use, the more energy you're producing and the faster you can go. How fast you're going when at your aerobic capacity is one of the best predictors of endurance performance. Consequently, we'll be discussing this topic a lot in this and the next few chapters, as it has much to do with how fit you are, regardless of age.

When you are at your aerobic capacity—maxed out and breathing really hard—you can maintain that level of effort only for a short time. This is true of all fit athletes, and it usually clocks in around 4 to 6 minutes, depending on your sport.[3] The less aerobically fit you are, the shorter the amount of time you can sustain such a high effort. The limiting factor is how much oxygen you can deliver to the working muscles and their capacity for using it. All of this amounts to a large portion of what we call "fitness."

Aerobic capacity is also known to many athletes by its scientific notation, "VO_2max." This is a shorthand way of expressing the definition of aerobic capacity: the maximal (max) volume (V) of oxygen (O_2) that the body can process during aerobic exercise. Just in case you're interested, the formula for it is:

VO_2max = milliliters of oxygen per kilogram of body weight per minute

Or more briefly:

$$VO_2max = mLO_2/kg/min$$

More simply put, VO_2max is how much oxygen you are capable of processing per minute relative to your weight. I'll come back to the weight portion later in this chapter.

The most accurate way to determine your VO_2max is to go to a facility that offers such testing. This could be a university physiology lab, a medical office, or a health club. Testing is also offered by some running, cycling, and triathlon retail stores and often by coaches. Since VO_2max varies by sport, you should be tested only in your sport, if possible. Because of all the equipment involved and the shortage of available venues, some sports, such as swimming, paddling, and Nordic skiing, are difficult to test. Facilities for such sport testing are available, but they are fewer in number than for running, cycling, and rowing. The testing is not cheap, so be sure to shop around. It's important that you find a facility with someone who has experience testing athletes, not just normal people. One more important point: Prepare for the test as if it were a race by resting for a couple of days beforehand. Fatigue will confound the results.

The technician will fit you with a mask that covers your nose and mouth in order to capture your breath. The typical test includes a warm-up followed by a steady, stepped progression of intensity every few minutes until you can't go any longer. When you hit that point, you've reached your

VO_2max. The air you exhale at this point is then analyzed to determine how much oxygen you used for a minute. Once the test is completed, you plug in your body weight, and the formula spits out your VO_2max. Pretty nifty.

World-class endurance athletes, both male and female, typically have VO_2max values in the 60s, 70s, and 80s, with females registering about 10 percent lower than males. That means these top-end athletes consume 60 to 80 milliliters of oxygen per kilogram of body weight per minute. (A milliliter is about two-tenths of a teaspoon, or 0.000264 gallons. So if a male athlete who weighs 154 pounds, or 70 kg, has a VO_2max of 70 mLO$_2$/kg/min, his body is effectively using about 1.3 gallons of oxygen in a minute at his top end. Note, though, that he's actually breathing in and out at least five times as much total gases in a minute, over 6.5 gallons, because air is composed mostly of nitrogen; oxygen accounts for only about 21 percent of the air we breathe, and some unused oxygen is exhaled.)

These are very big numbers when it comes to VO_2max. The highest numbers ever found by testing were of elite, male Nordic skiers, cyclists, runners, and rowers. Those numbers were in the 90s. The highest numbers for women fall into the upper 70s, a difference that is due primarily to a woman's lower ratio of lean muscle to overall body weight.

As for the effect of age, your VO_2max today is likely to be far less than it was when you were younger, even if you are a former world-class athlete. As we saw in Chapter 1, aerobic capacity declines with age, along with endurance performance.

A very rough way to estimate your VO_2max was developed by some Danish sport scientists in the early 2000s based on maximal and resting heart rates.[4] This formula is likely to give you a number that's off by a bit—perhaps quite a bit—but it can be remarkably close for some:

$$VO_2max = 15 \ (HRmax \div HRrest)$$

TABLE 3.1. **VO$_2$max by Age Group for Nonathletic Males and Females**

AGE	MALES	FEMALES
10–19	47–65	38–46
20–29	43–52	33–42
30–39	39–48	30–38
40–49	36–44	26–35
50–59	34–41	24–33
60–69	31–38	22–30
70–79	28–35	20–27

Source: Wilmore JH, Costill DL. 2005. *Physiology of Sport and Exercise*: 3rd Edition. Champaign, IL: Human Kinetics.

To use this formula, divide your *known* maximal heart rate (not the commonly used but highly inaccurate 220 minus your age), the highest you've seen in the past couple of years, by your resting heart rate, the lowest you've seen recently when fully rested. Multiply the result by 15. That's a very rough estimate of your VO$_2$max for the sport in which you measured HRmax.

How high can you get your aerobic capacity? Your VO$_2$max *potential* is largely dependent on who your parents were. This is a conclusion based on classic research showing that identical twins have nearly identical aerobic capacities.[5] It means you have a genetic ceiling, but don't get hung up on that—so does everyone. Instead, focus on the task at hand, which is to strive in your training to achieve a VO$_2$max as close to your maximum potential as possible. If you never work out at or near such a high intensity, your VO$_2$max is likely to decline at a faster rate than if you do. Again, that was what we saw in the longitudinal studies discussed in Chapter 1.

In case you do get tested and want to know what the numbers mean when compared with those for other similarly aged people, Table 3.1 lists some common VO$_2$max ranges for males and females ages 10 to 79 who were considered to be in "good" shape. Note that these are people selected from the general population. As a serious endurance athlete, your number will almost certainly be higher, probably by at least 10 percent and perhaps by as much as 50 percent.

Since aerobic capacity is closely related to age, the higher your number is relative to your age-group peers, the "younger" you are.[6] If you know your VO_2max, preferably from testing but perhaps from the above heart rate estimation method, find it in the appropriate column in Table 3.1 and look across to the "Age" column to find your "fitness" age group. Note that you will get only a rough estimate because the numbers in the rows overlap. But if you're looking for good news, you will almost surely find it in this table.

Moreover, as an athlete, your fitness age as represented by your VO_2max is probably a better indicator of your body's status than your chronological age. People with high aerobic capacities, and therefore lower fitness ages, are generally healthier and live longer.[7] When you find your "age" in this table, don't be surprised to find that you are years younger than you thought!

As I mentioned earlier, VO_2max varies somewhat by sport. This has to do with how much muscle is being used to propel the body and the effects of gravity and drag on effort. These differences raise the issue of what the various test results may be for an athlete who is proficient in several sports. For example, a triathlete's VO_2max is likely to be highest for running and lowest for swimming, with cycling in between. Running involves the use of bigger muscles and a greater effort to overcome gravity when compared with cycling and swimming. There could easily be a 10 percent range from highest to lowest, and possibly even more. So if your only sport is cycling, for example, it's important that you test in cycling, if that's at all possible, to get the most accurate result.

If you decide to be tested, you must also understand that endurance fitness, regardless of what specifically is measured, is known to vary throughout the season. To even out the effect of seasonal ups and downs on your VO_2max measurement, testing once each season at a standard time is a way of gauging how your fitness compares with that of previous years. For example, you may choose to test only at the end of a Base period in your training (see "Training Periodization" in Chapter 6). Some athletes who are very serious about precisely measuring their progress are tested several times in a season, but this is not necessary.

In fact, knowing your VO_2max is not necessary at all for training purposes. Testing is mostly useful for motivation and can be fun for bragging rights. Where it may help is in determining how great your effort should be when you do aerobic-capacity workouts, as I'll explain in Chapter 4. But you can figure that out without costly testing. I'll show you how later.

In actuality, the most valuable information you may glean from a VO_2max test has to do not with aerobic capacity but rather with your lactate threshold and how your body uses fat and carbohydrate to produce energy at various heart rates or intensities. Ask the test technician if all of these personal data can be explained to you after the test is over.

Lactate Threshold

Explaining lactate threshold often makes for a very long-winded and convoluted discussion, since it relies heavily on an understanding of exercise physiology. I'm going to try to keep it brief, and I will give you a couple of bail-out points along the way. But even if you have fought your way through it before, there is some new information about it that you may find interesting.

For starters, science uses several names to explain the various changes taking place in your body about the time you start to "redline" in an interval workout or a short, fast race. The accumulated changes at this rather high intensity result in a rapid increase in your breathing, the feeling that the effort is quite high and perhaps becoming unsustainable (around 6 or 7 on a 1 [low] to 10 [high] scale of perceived exertion), and perhaps even a burning sensation in the working muscles. Scientists may refer to what you are experiencing as the "anaerobic threshold," "lactate threshold," "maximum lactate steady state," or "onset of blood lactate accumulation," depending on how and when your redline effort is measured. All of these terms refer to that moment, slightly before to slightly after, when you experience this effort at an intensity level of approximately 7. While scientists debate the merits of using one of these terms as opposed to the others, we won't worry about semantics.

To further complicate the matter, there are two lactate thresholds. The first one occurs at a very low level of intensity, around what is also called the "aerobic threshold," which I'll explain in a later chapter. So if you do get tested for VO_2max and you want to know your lactate threshold—which you should—be sure that the technician discovers both of them. Since you'll likely be doing a gas-analysis test (wearing a mask and measuring oxygen) and not an actual lactate test (pricking the finger or ear to get a drop of blood in order to measure lactate concentrations), the technician will probably refer to what you want to know as the "anaerobic threshold." That's fine and saves some confusion. In this case, be sure to ask for your "aerobic threshold" as well. You'll use both thresholds in training, but the higher one is the more critical for our purposes.

I know it's all very confusing. It's the same way for scientists.[8]

You don't have to be an exercise physiologist to understand training, and you don't need expensive tests to train. I'll show you later how you can do field tests to find your VO_2max and both lactate thresholds. Nevertheless, it helps if you are familiar with what's going on inside your body when you experience the higher-intensity lactate threshold. So let's take an Exercise Physiology 101 short course. If you'd rather not dig into the science, feel free to skip ahead to the "Economy" section.

As your muscles use carbohydrate to create energy (specifically, they use glycogen—the muscle's form of stored sugar), they create a by-product inside the cells called lactic acid. As the intensity of your workout increases, this lactic acid begins to seep out of the muscle cell into the fluid in the surrounding space and into the bloodstream. (Remember osmosis from your high school chemistry or biology class?) As it seeps out, it changes its chemical composition and releases hydrogen ions. At this point, it is sometimes called "lactate." Despite its bad-boy reputation, left over from an incomplete understanding of its function, lactate is actually a beneficial substance for the body during exercise, as it is used to create more energy so that exercise may continue. In other words, lactate does *not* cause fatigue or muscle soreness, as is often claimed. Rather, it's hydrogen ions that are the real exercise bogeyman. The accumulation of hydrogen ions creates an acidic environment for the working muscles. This is what produces the burning sensation and labored breathing at high effort levels.

YOU DON'T HAVE to be an exercise physiologist to understand training, and you don't need expensive tests to train.

Measuring lactate levels in the blood is merely a convenient way of estimating the quantity of hydrogen ions in the body. The more intense the workout, the greater the amount of lactate released into the blood and the more hydrogen ions you have interfering with muscle contractions. At low intensities, below the lactate threshold, your body has no problem getting rid of the ions. But as you pass through your lactate threshold, they begin to accumulate, and you start breathing heavily. The purpose of the labored breathing is to remove hydrogen ions from the body, not to get more oxygen in. The other way the trained athlete copes with the hydro-gen ion buildup is by developing the ability to tolerate it. Essentially, you can become less sensitive to its negative effects by training at or near the upper lactate threshold.

Your heart rate, power, or pace at the moment when hydrogen ions begin accumulating is defined as your lactate threshold intensity. The higher your lactate threshold is as a percentage of your aerobic capacity, the more fit you are and the faster you will race, especially in steady-state events such as running races, triathlons, or cycling time trials.

It's common for fit athletes' lactate thresholds to occur at about 80 percent of their aerobic capacities. One athlete may have the same VO_2max as another but have a lower or higher lactate threshold as a percentage of VO_2max.[9] The higher it is, the faster and longer you can go hard. Although you may be able to sustain your aerobic capacity intensity only for a hand-ful of minutes, most well-conditioned athletes can sustain their lactate threshold (anaerobic threshold) for about an hour. The aerobic threshold (lower lactate threshold) can be held for several hours.

The 1-hour limit to the upper lactate threshold is so common that there is a new term to describe it. It was created by Hunter Allen and Dr. Andrew Coggan, the authors of *Training and Racing with a Power Meter*, and it eliminates all of the scientific mumbo jumbo. They call it "func-tional threshold."[10] This is the average bike power, or run, swim, row, or Nordic ski pace, that you can maintain for 1 hour. Simple. And it doesn't require understanding exercise physiology.

In addition to power and pace, we can apply this functional-threshold concept in another way. If you are using heart rate to determine your training zones, your Functional Threshold Heart Rate (FTHR) is your average heart rate for a 1-hour race effort. How easy is that? This is unique to the sport, so your rowing, Nordic skiing, swimming, cycling, and running FTHRs are likely to be different. Therefore, your heart rate zones will also be unique to each sport. We'll come back to the functional threshold to explain how you can use a field test to determine it and then apply the results to your training and racing.

Economy

The last of the three physiological fitness determiners is economy. We know less about economy than about aerobic capacity and lactate threshold, but it may be the most important of the three. It has to do with how efficiently you use oxygen while exercising.

As we saw in the earlier aerobic-capacity discussion, measuring the oxygen you use during exercise is the way in which we measure how much energy is expended, since both oxygen and stored fuel (primarily fat or glycogen) are needed to power your muscles. This is similar to how your car works, although what is being measured differs. A car blends oxygen with stored fuel (the gasoline in the tank) to make the engine go. To calculate a car's efficiency, we measure the gas it burns instead of the oxygen it uses because measuring the gasoline is easy. In our bodies, while it is not so easy to measure the fat and glycogen used in exercise, it is relatively easy to measure oxygen uptake, so that's what we use when testing the human engine.

Also, as with a car, your body has an economy rating. For a car, we call it miles per gallon. For your body, it's expressed as milliliters of oxygen per minute, which is nothing more than the VO_2max formula minus the body-weight part. The less oxygen you use per minute at a given submaximal pace or power, the more economical you are. The more economical you are, the less energy (fat and glycogen) it takes to move your body. If you're running a 100-meter sprint, conserving energy is not a big deal. You have plenty of stored energy for such a short duration. But if you're running a marathon, competing in an Ironman triathlon, or racing 100 miles on your bike or skis, economy is huge. This has to due with resistance to fatigue. You don't want to waste energy at such long distances.

An athlete can have a relatively low aerobic capacity yet be quite competitive if he or she has an excellent economy. The 1970s marathon runner Frank Shorter is an excellent example. He was reported to have a VO_2max of 72. As you'll recall from our earlier discussion of aerobic capacity, that's rather low for a world-class male runner; most are in the upper 70s, with some in the 80s and higher. Shorter, however, won the 1972 Olympic Games marathon gold medal and the silver medal at the 1976 Games. (He probably should have won the gold in 1976, too, as the winner, Waldemar Cierpinski of East Germany, was later implicated in doping.) Between 1971 and 1976, Shorter was ranked either first or second in the world for the marathon every year. During his career, he won several big races, including four wins at Japan's Fukuoka Marathon, which was generally considered the most prestigious in the world at the time. Shorter was one of the most economical runners ever studied.[11] He made the most of his "low" VO_2max because he simply didn't waste any energy.

Just as aerobic capacity has a genetic component, economy is also determined to some extent by who your parents are.[12] For example, we know that being tall with long arms and big feet and hands improves economy in swimming (think Michael Phelps). In cycling, having a long thigh bone relative to your total leg length improves economy. For running, being of small stature with a long shin bone is a winning economy combination (think of the Kenyans who currently dominate the sport).

In addition, for endurance athletes in general, economy is improved by having a high percentage of slow-twitch muscle fibers. The count of your mitochondria, the little powerhouses in the muscle cell that produce energy, is also important. These are all things over which we have little or no control but which have a significant impact on our oxygen use per minute.

Age also affects economy. Children are not as economical as adults, but as they age, their economy improves.[13] In a similar way, the longer you've been seriously training in your sport, the more economical you are likely to have become. That's largely due to the body adapting in order to conserve energy. All of this implies that aging and experience may actually have a beneficial effect when it comes to this important predictor of performance. That's one point for us oldsters.

With this as a prelude, what things can you control to improve your economy so that you use fewer milliliters of oxygen per minute? Perhaps the most common factor is technique. You can change how you move in order to waste less energy. You must realize that if you decide to go this route and make changes in your current technique, there will be a period during which you will become less efficient. This will show up as a higher-than-normal heart rate and somewhat more labored breathing at any given speed or power. And it may take weeks, if not months, to make the new technique your normal one. At that point, you should be faster at the same heart rates as before.

THE LONGER you've been seriously training in your sport, the more economical you are likely to have become.

Then again, you may not. One thing is clear when you study technique as a marker of economy: You can't count on it to improve performance. Studies of runners who change their running technique to supposedly become more economical often experience no improvement. Some become less economical in the long term, even if they see a short-term improvement.[14] This just confirms why economy remains such a great mystery to sport scientists.

But there are other factors that are generally beneficial for economy across nearly all endurance sports. First among these is reducing excess body weight. Another is using lighter equipment. For example, biomechanics experts have shown that every additional 100 grams (3.5 ounces) of running-shoe weight increases the oxygen cost of running by some-where between 1 and 2 percent.[15] There are several other sport-specific efficiency improvers. Perhaps the most notable is aerobars on a time trial or triathlon bike along with other aerodynamic equipment such as wheels, helmet, and bike frame.

As a swimmer, you may improve economy by improving the flexibility of your shoulders, knees, and ankles, especially the ability to point your toes.[16] Interestingly, the research shows that having *less* flexibility in the ankle joint, the opposite of what we are usually led to believe, makes for more economical running, as this appears to improve the release of energy stored in your calf muscle with each foot strike.[17] When it comes to econ-omy, the results that deliver improvement are often counterintuitive.

Of the three training components—duration, intensity, and frequency—the one that many believe may do the least to improve economy is dura-tion. Going long to the point of fatigue often causes a breakdown in tech-nique and therefore economy. Frequency, while not scientifically confirmed, and intensity may prove much more beneficial. In terms of how often you train, one way to improve your technique and possibly your economy is to practice your sport often even if each session is brief. For example, a time-restricted athlete with only 2 hours a week to devote to training could pursue improvements in economy by working out four times a week for 30 minutes each time. That schedule may not be best for endurance but may improve economy faster than doing two 1-hour work-outs each week.

There are studies showing that high-intensity training is more beneficial for economy than low-intensity.[18] To improve your economy (or perhaps even to maintain it), train frequently and include high-intensity workouts. Of course, you're probably already training quite often, and intensity is a tool that we will return to several times in the following chapters.

There are some training modes that may also prove beneficial. For example, plyometric exercises have been shown to improve economy in runners and cyclists.[19] Plyometric exercise involves explosive jumping, bounding, and hopping drills. There is still a great deal of debate about whether or not traditional strength training with weights improves economy. Some studies show improvement for several sports,[20] whereas others have found no performance or economy enhancement.[21] I believe strength training does contribute to improvement, but not for all athletes. I've coached many athletes over the years with initial signs of inadequate strength, and I've seen them improve their performances remarkably after a winter of lifting weights, provided they did exercises that closely mimic the movements of their sport. (I'll get into all of this in Chapter 4.)

Interestingly, a very high VO_2max and excellent economy have never been reported to co-occur in the same athlete, at least among elite athletes who have been the subjects of such studies—and there have been many.[22] For them, and possibly for all of us, one's greater physiological asset is either aerobic capacity or economy, but not both. This explains Frank Shorter, and probably you, too. There's a great likelihood that you are much better in one of these two fitness markers than in the other. It's not known why. Another economy mystery.

What's Limiting Your Fitness?

So that's it. There are just three things that define endurance fitness. *Everything* you do in training is related to one or more of them. Stretching? Economy. Long workouts? Aerobic capacity. Intervals? Aerobic capacity, lactate threshold, and economy. Weight lifting? Economy. Muscular endurance? Lactate threshold. And so on. All workouts fit neatly into one or more of these three categories. So training to become more fit really isn't all that complex. The biggest issue is deciding where your limiters lie and then designing workouts around one or more of these three in order to improve them.

So what do the people in white lab coats have to say about these three in regard to aging? Of the three, they tell us that the most common marker of age-related performance decline is aerobic capacity. Lactate threshold follows a distant second. Economy is an even more distant third because economy seems to remain stable over time.[23] That economy would not be a good age-related performance predictor makes sense; after all, after decades of training and racing, the movement patterns of older athletes have become well honed.[24] So it's most likely aerobic capacity that we need to examine closely to see what might be expected as the candles on the birthday cake increase.

I say "most likely" because every athlete is an individual, and your limiter might not be aerobic capacity. It could well be lactate threshold or economy. These are just less likely to be the reason that your performance is heading south.

Now that we're up to speed on what fitness is, let's go back to all of aging's big three limiters to see if we can figure out what is holding you back and what can be done about it. In quick review from earlier in this chapter, they are:

- Decreasing aerobic capacity
- Increasing body fat
- Shrinking muscles

Decreasing Aerobic Capacity

As mentioned before, sports scientists generally consider this the most likely culprit to explain the decrease in performance with advancing age.[25]

TABLE 3.2. **Aging and VO₂max in Fit Male Cyclists**

AGE GROUP	VO₂MAX (AVERAGE)	% CHANGE
20–29	69.5	—
30–39	64.2	–7.6
40–49	65.0	+1.2
50–59	62.7	–3.5
60–69	43.6	–30.5
70–79	36.8	–15.6

Source: F. B. Wyatt and J. P. McCarthy, "Ventilatory Parameters Influence the Decline in VO₂max in Fit Male Cyclists," presentation at the 4th American Society of Exercise Physiologists Annual Meeting, June 2001, Memphis, TN.

You simply aren't as capable of delivering oxygen to your working muscles and using it as effectively as when you were younger, and the decline is likely to continue at an increasing rate with each passing year. Table 3.2 illustrates what one cross-sectional research study found happened to the aerobic capacities of fit male cyclists.

You may well be doing something to turn this around, but my experience has been that most aging athletes aren't. The key to maintaining your aerobic capacity is our old friend high-intensity training. By age 50, most athletes are starting to cut back on such workouts. And it's no secret why: They're hard, and they often have negative side effects such as an increased risk of injury (we'll look at how to avoid this in Chapter 4). By the time we're in our 60s, high intensity probably feels like a thing of the past, seldom to be revisited. Just as we saw with most of the athletes in the longitudinal studies discussed in Chapter 1, most of us steadily gravitate toward long, slow distance as the focus of our workouts.

But perhaps aerobic capacity isn't your limiter. If, as a result of past and recent testing, you are known to have a high VO₂max for your age that has been maintained at well under 1 percent of decline yearly, then we can conclude that aerobic capacity more than likely isn't your limiter.[26] It's either lactate threshold or economy. Given that economy is seldom a limiter for seniors, we could further deduce that lactate threshold is the culprit. Again, this appears to be rare for the senior athlete, as lactate threshold, as a percent of aerobic capacity, tends to increase with age among athletes.[27]

So what should you do in training? That's the subject of Chapter 4. For now, I want you to get a good handle on what is causing your decline in aerobic capacity so that you will be better prepared to manage all aspects of your lifestyle (nurture). Doing so will produce positive changes in your fitness physiology. I hope this will also help you realize that the solution is at least 99.9 percent training, diet, and lifestyle and not some device, potion, or pill you find advertised in the back of a magazine. There are a ton of these quick fixes, all "guaranteed" to improve your aerobic capacity. Pay no attention. They won't. If they worked as advertised, they would be banned. All they can do with any certainty is lighten your wallet. The key for nearly all senior athletes is high intensity blended with other effective types of training, including adequate recovery, along with a diet and lifestyle that promote high performance.

All of these topics will be addressed in coming chapters. For now, let's return to understanding what's happening to your body that results in aerobic capacity being the most likely limiter for your performance decline in recent years. This involves understanding a bit of aging exercise physiology—how your senior body works during training and competition.

There are two major subsystems of aerobic capacity—oxygen delivery and oxygen uptake. The delivery of oxygen to the muscles involves your lungs, heart, blood, arteries, and capillaries. On the uptake side, the muscles must grab the oxygen as it flows past in the capillaries, pull it in, and use it to produce energy. This is the work of the aerobic enzymes found in a muscle's cells. Once inside the muscle, the oxygen is combined with fat

Endurance Exercise and Your Heart

LARRY
CRESWELL,
MD

In recent years, considerable media attention has been paid to the deaths of middle-aged endurance athletes during triathlons and long-distance running races. I'm thankful that these incidents are rare. We've also learned from scientific reporting about unusual fibrosis, or scarring, as well as calcium buildup in the coronary arteries of seemingly healthy longtime runners. Although these findings have raised concerns, their implications truly remain unknown. It isn't surprising, then, that I frequently get questions about the safety of endurance sports for athletes older than 50 years.

My general advice is that strenuous endurance training is both safe and beneficial for serious veteran athletes, particularly if due consideration is given to the athlete's heart health. We should remember that the many health benefits of exercise are well established for young and veteran athletes alike. Not only does exercise improve our overall health, it also extends our life expectancy. For many reasons, exercise should be part of everybody's routine. This is particularly true for older individuals. Many professional organizations now recommend 150 minutes of exercise per week, regardless of age. We also know that including some high-intensity exercise may increase the health and longevity benefits derived from exercise.

Not surprisingly, though, exercise places extra demands on the heart. For athletes of any age, unrecognized heart disease can pose some risk. For instance, unrecognized conditions can sometimes damage the heart over a period of years because of extra workload placed on the heart. This process is insidious. Or there may be a sudden problem such as heart attack, aortic rupture, or even sudden cardiac death. Both types of risk deserve attention from the veteran athlete. It's important not to overlook latent heart disease.　　　　»

Continued

In younger individuals, our concern centers around congenital (inherited) heart conditions, such as "holes" in the heart, abnormal development of the coronary arteries, electrical problems such as the long Q-T syndrome, or hypertrophic cardiomyopathy. Most of these conditions manifest in athletes during their first three decades of life.

For veteran athletes, our concern turns to the development of coronary artery disease (CAD)—blockages in the coronary arteries, which bring blood flow and oxygen to the heart muscle itself. That process occurs slowly over decades and is related to a set of risk factors that includes a family history of CAD, high blood pressure, diabetes, smoking, elevated blood lipid levels, and simply increasing age.

I recommend that veteran athletes partner with their doctors on two fronts. First, you should visit your doctor periodically for a heart-focused checkup and for ongoing assessments of your risk of CAD. You should monitor your risk factors and modify those that can be changed for the better. Additional testing such as a stress test makes sense for those at moderate risk. Second, you should take warning signs seriously. Problems such as chest pain or discomfort, unusual shortness of breath, light-headedness or blacking out, palpitations, and unusual fatigue should be investigated promptly.

or glycogen, resulting in a muscular contraction. This is quite a complex mechanism, and the demise of any of the subsystems could account for a decrease in your aerobic capacity.

Of the two subsystems, delivery is generally considered the one most likely to be the major contributor to a decline in aerobic capacity.[28] And the common reasons for that, when it comes to senior athletes, are most commonly thought to be decreases in stroke volume and maximum heart rate.[29] Stroke volume is the amount of blood pumped with each beat of the heart.

It is largely dependent on the size and contractility of the heart's left ventricle, the chamber that pumps blood out to the body. Older people in general tend to have larger left ventricles than young people, and in aging athletes it's even larger than among those who are sedentary.[30] But as with any muscle, if the left ventricle is seldom challenged to pump a lot of blood per beat, size and contractility may be lost, resulting in a decrease in aerobic capacity.[31] This seems to be more common in men than in women.[32]

The reduction in max heart rate with aging is also often thought to contribute to the decline in aerobic capacity,[33] as heart rate is generally believed to decrease by about one beat per year of life (hence the overused and wildly inaccurate formula "220 minus age"). Again, it appears that this may not be the case for women athletes who maintain the volume of their training despite growing older and experiencing the onset of menopause.[34] And to further confuse the matter, one longitudinal study of 15 well-trained male endurance athletes conducted 8 years after the initial testing found no change in maximal heart rate, yet their aerobic capacities declined by just slightly more than half a percent per year.[35] Their average age at the follow-up was 62. As with the women subjects in the previous study, the best predictor of the men's rates of loss of aerobic capacity was changes in training. Their training volume decreased about 20 percent on average over the 8 years from ages 54 to 62, and the average training intensity dropped by 7 to 10 percent. Only one of the subjects maintained both volume and intensity for the entire 8 years. He lost no aerobic capacity and improved his race performances. This is the guy whom we want to emulate as best we can.

So the jury is still out on exactly what the reasons may be for the drop in aerobic capacity that we experience with aging. As is often the case with all such matters related to performance and age, the exact causes are undoubtedly the result of many small changes taking place in your body over a lifetime.[36] Besides possible changes in stroke volume and max heart rate, the causes could have to do with slight changes in lung capacity, breathing muscles, the oxygen-carrying power of the blood, blood-vessel elasticity, capillary density, energy-producing mitochondria, and aerobic enzymes in the muscles. The only conclusions we can draw with some certainty are that aerobic capacity will continue to decline with age and that continuing to train your aerobic capacity, despite age, is likely to pay off by slowing, halting, or perhaps even temporarily reversing the decline. Again, the training solution for this aerobic-capacity dilemma is the subject of the next chapter.

Increasing Body Fat

Remember the formula for VO_2max, what I've been calling aerobic capacity throughout this chapter? Just in case, here it is again:

$$VO_2max = mLO_2/kg/min$$

The "mLO_2" (milliliters of oxygen) stands for how much oxygen you consume per minute (min) while exercising at a sustained, maximal intensity for several minutes.

Then there's that pesky "kg" in the formula. Now is finally the time to look at it more closely. It may have a lot to do with aerobic capacity decline over time as you age even if you maintain stroke volume, max heart rate, and everything else that potentially affects VO_2max. It refers to your body weight in kilograms. And since it's a denominator in the formula, meaning we divide by it, it has an inverse relationship to VO_2max. What this implies is that if your body weight increases (a higher kg), then your VO_2max decreases. So what? Well, it's a big deal. This isn't just some obscure, scientific formula that has little to do with the real world.

It's a problem because if you gain weight, the primary muscles that move you during training and racing have to work harder just to maintain the same pace you were capable of at a lower body weight when you were younger. How about we do a mental experiment to give this a real-world meaning?

Let's assume for this experiment that you are a runner, and we have you do two tests. Each involves running as fast as you can for 1 mile on a track. We'll give you a couple of days of recovery between the two sessions. For one of the test miles, you run wearing a backpack containing a 10-pound weight. For the other mile, you run just as you are—no weighted backpack. What might we expect the outcomes to be? It's obvious, isn't it? When wearing the extra 10 pounds, you'll run more slowly than you will unweighted. Why? Because you had to work harder carrying the extra weight. It doesn't matter if the extra weight is rocks in a backpack or excess body fat. The outcome is the same: Your VO_2max drops quite a bit.

IF YOUR SPORT is dependent on performance relative to gravity, then gaining weight is likely a problem.

We could have done the experiment with you as a Nordic skier or a cyclist climbing a long hill. In fact, we could have used any sport in which gravity plays a significant role in how fast the athlete goes. The other side of this coin is that the extra weight is not as significant for sports in which gravity plays a small role—swimming, for example, or racing a bike on a flat surface. Extra weight, in the form of muscle or perhaps even body fat, may prove to be an advantage in such sports. Open-water swimmers often try to put on a little more body fat before a long open-water swim to serve as insulation against cold water. Cyclists with huge thigh muscles may be really fast when it comes to flat time trials, but they are seldom good at climbing in the mountains.

The bottom line is this: If your sport is dependent on performance relative to gravity, then gaining weight is likely a problem.[37]

Of course, you may gain body fat while losing muscle (a matter I'll come back to in the next section) and therefore not gain weight. Muscle is denser, and thus muscle weighs more than fat at any given size. So losing a little bit of lean muscle while putting on some blubber and thus keeping your body weight constant may have the same negative effect on VO$_2$max. Muscle can contribute to how fast you go in a race, whereas fat is nothing but an anchor that must be dragged along.

What we're really talking about is body composition—how much lean body mass you have versus how much fat. With some exceptions, as noted earlier, endurance athletes perform best with a low percentage of body fat.

As you probably know, however, with advancing age comes a noticeable shift away from leanness and toward more flab. In the normal population, there is a significant change in body composition starting around age 65.[38] Compared with where they were at age 25, by their late 60s most men have lost about 26 pounds of lean mass and women about 11 pounds—mostly muscle.[39]

Less is known about the relationship between serious exercise and lean body mass changes with age, but it appears that exercise is beneficial for maintaining muscle while limiting gains in body fat.[40] So we might expect that serious athletes, including those in their late 60s and beyond, would experience less change in their body composition than sedentary folks.[41] But when it comes to performance, how you compare with your nonexercising neighbors is of no consequence. If you are adding fat and losing muscle, your racing will suffer.

Even as aging athletes, we can expect some change in body composition—more fat and less lean. What's causing this shift, especially the "more fat" portion? It has to do, in large part, with an enzyme called lipoprotein lipase (LPL). As we age, LPL results in an accumulation of adipose tissue, what we call "love handles," wherever it is found in the body. This is a rather complex activity related to insulin sensitivity and your normal diet,[42] which we'll examine more closely in Chapter 8.

With aging, we can expect an increase in fat deposits wherever LPL is found in abundance in the body.[43] In men, when younger, testosterone keeps LPL from being very active and helps maintain body leanness. But less testosterone is produced with age, and so LPL is less restricted. The result is an accumulation of fat on certain sites around the body where it is abundant, especially the belly. Women throughout life have active LPL primarily on the hips and butt, so when younger, they store fat in those locations. But following menopause, LPL becomes more prolific on the abdomen, resulting in fat storage there also.

Closely related to the issue of weight gain, which is actually fat accumulation, is the matter of dwindling muscles. That's where we're going next.

Shrinking Muscles

The previous section on weight gain let the cat out of the bag on this topic. It showed that there is a change in body composition with aging that results from the interplay of two factors: an increase in body fat and a decrease in muscle. Along with the decline in aerobic capacity discussed earlier, these body fat and muscle changes make up the big three most common reasons for the decline in performance as we get older.

Let's start by once again looking at the bad news when it comes to muscle and aging. In Chapter 4 I'll stop telling you about all of these negative consequences of growing old and get on with what can be done about them. But for now, you need to understand what you're up against.

Sarcopenia is the loss of muscle as normal people age.[44] Here's what science currently knows about it. Starting around age 40, a progressive decrease of muscle begins. At first there appears to be a loss of well under 1 percent per year, but the rate accelerates as the years pile up. By age 70, the average, sedentary person has lost about 24 percent of his or her muscle mass. Then the slope gets even more slippery. After age 70, the rate of loss increases to about 1.5 to 2 percent per year, so that by age 80, an additional 15 to 20 percent of muscle is gone. That explains why many senescent people look so frail.

The loss of muscle is due largely to a decrease in hormone production that parallels the fate of your muscles.[45] By age 40, testosterone production is beginning to drop, contributing to significant losses of muscle in men.[46] In women, estrogen also takes a nosedive with a similar (though not as great) change in women's muscles.[47] Likewise, growth hormone and insulinlike growth factor, two other hormones tied closely to muscle maintenance and development, also go into decline as you move north of 40. As explained earlier, this loss of muscle may not be apparent on the bathroom scale because there is an increase in body fat at the same time.

All of this may apply only to your sedentary neighbor. Less is known about the effect of age on the muscles of serious endurance athletes like you. But we know something about this, and for once, the news isn't so bad.

A couple of recent, unique studies from the University of Western Ontario lend support to the "use it or lose it" concept.[48] The researchers counted the number of motor units in recreationally active young (about age 25) subjects, old (about age 65) runners, and old (about age 65) sedentary subjects. A motor unit is a group of muscle fibers activated by a single nerve. With normal, or sedentary, aging, which has a large disuse component, those nerves die, and their associated muscle fibers atrophy, and so inactive older folks lose muscle size, strength, and power quite rapidly.

This has been known for some time based on studies of aging rats and has been confirmed for humans by this study. But how about the study's athletes? How did their motor units do?

Basically, the researchers found that as endurance athletes, we're a bit different. Runners in their 60s had about the same number of motor units in their tibialis anterior (a shin muscle) as did the young subjects. But when they counted the motor units in sedentary but healthy people also in their 60s, the scientists discovered that the inactive older folks had 35 percent fewer motor units than the same-age runners. Essentially, the old runners still had young leg muscles. That's great news, for a change. But there's more.

The Canadian researchers logically wondered if this finding meant that *all* the muscle motor units in an aging runner's body were maintained or just the running-related motor units. In a follow-up study, they counted motor units in the biceps brachii (upper arm) of aging runners, young subjects, and the aging sedentary.[49] They found that the older runners had about 48 percent fewer motor units in their arms than did the young runners and about the same as the older sedentary. Apparently, exercise does not maintain muscles unless they are strenuously trained. So there is now little doubt: Use it or lose it. Right?

MANY OF WHAT we consider to be the inevitable changes of aging are things that we have some control over.

Before we do cartwheels, we need to ask whether this result could be the consequence of who the subjects were. After all, this was a cross-sectional study; the subjects may have self-selected. People who maintained their motor units may have continued to compete into old age, whereas those who didn't maintain them for whatever reason may have dropped out of their sport at a much younger age. I wish we could take a look at some longitudinal studies of aging and motor units to see if these results hold true when athletes are followed for several years. Unfortunately, such research doesn't exist. Sorry to introduce this sour note, but it's important that we differentiate facts from speculation.

A related issue, one that's critical to our purpose here, has to do with reversibility. If muscle has been lost, can it be regained? Chances are that it can be, but the later in life one waits to start the muscle rebuilding, the more limited the results are likely to be. Muscle growth is still possible even at a well-advanced age. For example, a study out of Tufts University in Medford, Massachusetts, had 80 previously inactive subjects, ages 70 to 85, do resistance training for 6 months.[50] Their muscle mass improved by 1.3 percent by the end of the study. All of this apparently has to do with those stem cells discussed back in Chapter 2.

There was also one interesting twist on the outcome of the Tufts study among the aging subjects. Those who experienced the greatest improvement in muscle gain (1.3 percent) also took in more protein by using a supplement throughout the study. Those who didn't take in extra protein increased their muscle mass by only about half as much (0.6 percent). Let's file that away for later use and see if other research found the same thing.

We're starting to pull a lot of pieces together on the subject of shrinking muscles. My take on all of it is this: The primary cause of the decline in muscle with aging is most likely lack of use—an increasingly sedentary lifestyle as we get older. What I'm suggesting, with increasing support from science, is that nurture, not nature, is responsible for most of this loss.[51] Nature, of course, still plays a role and should not be summarily dismissed.[52] As we age, muscle is lost for both reasons. But nurture is something we can control, and as athletes, we are in a better place than most to minimize the loss of muscle.

This trend toward a less vigorous lifestyle happens even in serious senior athletes. It seems that as athletes grow older, their training becomes less strenuous. There may be lots of good reasons for that; injury avoidance is certainly one of them. Regardless, reducing intensity can and does result in a decrease in muscle, including the muscles that are most important to movement in your sport. In Chapter 4 I'll tell you what can be done in training to increase hormone production to help with the rebuilding of dwindling muscles, and in Chapter 8 I'll come back to examine protein intake and aging muscles.

Over the Hill?

I know what you're thinking, and I agree: There wasn't much in the way of good news in this chapter. Unfortunately, there's even more to the downside of aging that's been left unexplored. It's not just decreasing aerobic capacity, increasing body fat, and shrinking muscles that affect our performance as we age. While these may be the common big three limiters when it comes to performance with aging, there's more happening in our bodies that we need to understand in order to counteract the negative effects. These include the loss of bone density, an increasing propensity for total-body acidity, a slowing of the metabolism, a loss of joint range of motion, and more. We may also include other changes that senior athletes often experience, such as an increased risk of injury and a weakened immune system that makes them more susceptible to disease. These latter changes can result in a decreased training load and a big and rather sudden drop in fitness that may not be fully reclaimed once healthy again.

The magnitude of the impact on your performance of all of this results from the interplay of nature and nurture in your life. You can't control the nature part. But as I've pointed out many times in these first three chapters, many of what we consider to be the inevitable changes of aging are essentially the result of things that we have some degree of control over—how we nurture our bodies.

If you decide you have some degree of control over your destiny as a senior athlete, then you are taking the first step toward improved race performances. Aging is first and foremost an attitude. Whether you decide you're over the hill or not, you're right.

FASTER STRONGER LEANER!

In Part II, we present solutions to the problems identified in Part I by examining how you can modify your training and lifestyle to improve performance in your sport. These solutions come from sport science and from my experience as a lifelong athlete, a coach for more than three decades, and a 70-year-old man who wants to continue high-performance training and racing. I'm confident that I have the same concerns about aging that you have. I'll tell you what I've learned and what I think are the solutions to the questions of aging posed in Part I. By the end of Part II, you should have the information you'll need to design a training and lifestyle plan that slows, or even temporarily reverses, the common ravages of age that cause the decline in performance for senior athletes.

THE HIGH-PERFORMANCE SENIOR ATHLETE

Age is whatever you think it is. You are as old as you think you are.

—MUHAMMAD ALI

There's no question that aging is a blend of genetics and lifestyle—nature and nurture. No one knows the exact proportions of these two factors—60-40, 70-30, or something else. Nor do we yet know for certain which has the most to do with how we age. What we do know is that research currently points to lifestyle—nurture—as having the greater effect. Leyk and associates at the German Sport University in Cologne summed it up pretty well: Aging is a "biological process that can be considerably speeded up or slowed down by multiple lifestyle-related factors."[1] In fact, every research study on aging agrees that lifestyle has a big impact on biology and largely determines your physiological age. That's important information because lifestyle—specifically our approach to training—is something we can control.

So what can you do in training to slow aging while maintaining or even improving fitness and performance? The answer is not all that difficult.

What drives the physiology of training for high performance when you are old is no different from what it was when you were 30 years younger. The principles of training don't change.

What does change is your capacity—physical and psychological—to handle the stresses associated with focused and serious workouts. And that's where we're headed in this chapter. We'll first try to determine your potential as an athlete. Can you improve, or are you already close to your limit? The remainder of the chapter will offer training advice based on sports science research to help you answer the athlete's most important question: What should I do in training?

Given that you are an experienced athlete who has been in your sport for a long time—perhaps for decades—I'm not going to suggest a completely new and detailed training schedule for you. Instead, in this and the next three chapters I will introduce ways you can tweak your training routine in order to get more speed and power out of your aging body and take race performance to a new and higher level.

Your Potential for High Performance

Goal-focused and challenging workouts are key to your success as an endurance athlete. Simply knowing this will not make it happen, however. You must actually do something about it by training as high-performance athletes train, albeit with age-related adjustments. High-performance training demands physical stress. As we age, we sometimes seek to avoid that stress. The pain of a hard workout exceeds mere discomfort—it hurts. It can also result in sore muscles and joints and even injuries. So it's not surprising that we often gradually shift our training from high intensity to long, slow distance (LSD) over the course of many years. That has consequences for performance.

Recall from Bruce Dill's and Michael Pollock's longitudinal studies described in Chapter 1 that the apparent reason some athletes experience a large decline in performance over time is their lack of hard training; they reduce the volume and intensity of their workouts, especially the intensity. Among aging athletes, there is all too often a tendency to lighten the training load. This can happen without your even being aware of it. Over several years, you may find that you've changed how you train, with the workload gradually shifting away from the volume and intensity of your younger days. Look back at your training logs from 10 years ago. It's likely you'll discover that you don't train as much or as intensely. Regardless of how your current training came about, if you have high-performance goals, a daily diet of easy workouts won't get the job done. It takes a great commitment to quality training to achieve at a high level in sport.

Later in this chapter, we will get into the topic of how to adjust workout intensity for age to improve performance. Chapter 6 discusses how to periodize your training to optimize both volume and intensity relative to age. But first we need to examine your commitment to serious training. Training to perform better, whatever that may mean for you, starts in your head.

Set Your Goal

What can you achieve in your sport? The first part of the answer is self-evaluation, followed by establishing a goal. I won't go into all the goal-setting stuff you've read and heard about for years and years, such as how a goal should be measurable, well defined, time oriented, and so on. You know all this, I'm sure. Instead, let's do something different: Let's look at goal setting as a function of age and, especially, potential.

The starting place for improved training and therefore better fitness is a well-considered goal based on what your aging body (and mind) is capable of achieving. Aiming for the stars sounds good when talking with your training buddies, but that usually means low commitment because deep down, you know the goal isn't possible. Be realistic and honest with yourself. I'd rather see you set a goal you know is achievable and then, later on, once imminent success becomes apparent, take it up another notch. That's far better than starting too high and later on losing motivation to continue toward the impossible.

REGARDLESS OF AGE, most of us are capable of achieving a great deal more than we even imagine is possible.

On the other hand, don't dumb down your expectations by assuming that you are incapable of achieving a high level of performance simply because of the number of years you've been on the planet. Regardless of age, most of us are capable of achieving a great deal more than we even imagine is possible.

Reaching your goal requires commitment. You must fully commit if you are to succeed. That means everything in your lifestyle needs to be in alignment with the goal. "Everything" includes the big things such as training, nutrition, and sleep, but it also embraces the less obvious such as whom you hang out with and their attitudes toward your goal.

Setting a reasonable goal raises a key self-evaluation question: What am I capable of achieving? I'm often asked in random e-mails from athletes (whom I know nothing about) what their potential is. I'm afraid my crystal ball doesn't work that way. There is no sure way of accurately knowing exactly what anyone's potential is. But because you know yourself better than anyone else, you can get a ballpark answer. It requires looking backward before projecting forward.

The more challenging and structured your training has been in recent years and the more dedicated you've been to working out, the less room

Senior Moment

LISA RAINSBERGER

Elite runners at the height of their professional running careers may never feel satisfied with a PR or race victory (I never did). Senior athletes often display the same dissatisfaction and complain about how "slow" they feel or comment on how they do not run as fast as they did a few years back. When I hear such talk, I worry. I worry about the senior athlete chasing PRs from the past at a rate that could lead to injury or a continued feeling of dissatisfaction.

I wish I had allowed myself to feel a bit more joy in my own past accomplishments. It is funny, but winning an age-group medal today feels almost as good as when I won the Chicago Marathon. A big difference is that I have more time these days to relish the victory before I rush off to the next race.

Elite runners set high standards, a habit that is hugely important to their success. Senior athletes can live and train with a similar mind-set of setting goals and reaching training and performance standards. However, senior athletes must also be mindful of "What can I do?" versus "What I used to do." As our bodies age (I am currently 52 years old), the training and racing days of years gone by should be a fond memory and not a template of how we try to train today.

When I hear a senior athlete make a self-deprecating comment about how slow they are or how they used to train, I try to steer them back to who they are now. I caution them to focus forward and not to use the past as the template for the future. I gently remind the senior athletes I coach that I will never set a new PR; I will most likely never again win a race or break a record; and I, too, now run races an hour or more slower than I used to! But do I still love to run, to race, to train? Yes! What differs is how I view who I am at the moment. Some races I am a tired soccer mom just clinging to 5 hours of sleep a night. Other times I am the »

Continued

athlete who just moved up an age group and will enter a race to try to win some hardware. And sometimes I cheer from the sidelines as I nurse an injury.

I think the hardest part of being an aging athlete is letting go of the past performances and training programs and figuring out who you are now. Once you move into the present and work with what you've got (not what you used to be), you will find the same moments of accomplishment, joy, and success that you had in years gone by. Just be sure to allow yourself to enjoy the moment before you move on to the next goal.

you have to get faster. But if you've been slacking—missing workouts or doing mostly LSD training—then there are probably a great many improvements you can make in the years ahead despite your age—*if* you set a realistic goal and fully commit to it.

What's realistic? In timed events such as swimming, running, triathlon, and bike time trials, if your best performances have slowed by more than 15 percent in the past decade, for whatever reason, and you are currently healthy, then I fully expect that you are capable of achieving at a much higher level. On the other hand, if your times have slowed by 5 percent or less in a decade, you may be quite close to your potential (and congratulations on your strong commitment to excellence!). Within this rather broad range is anyone's guess, but the closer your times are to a 15 percent drop, the more room you have to get fast again.

For most athletes, regardless of age, the greatest obstacle to better performance is psychological, not physiological. Your head needs to say yes. Most people simply lack the motivation to do what it takes. This can happen at any age, of course. Being 50 or 60 or 70 doesn't mean you have a pass to train more easily and yet somehow perform well. Patting yourself on the back for merely finishing or accomplishing other low goals will only hurt your shoulder, not make you faster. High performance has been and always will be based on hard work. That brings us back to volume and intensity.

You aren't old until age becomes your excuse. If you continue to remind yourself of your age and use it as a crutch, no matter what that number is, you'll come to believe that high achievement is impossible. That's probably the way your parents saw the world. Mine did. In my parents' day, after a certain age you weren't expected to do anything strenuous. Gardening and a walk around the block was about as tough as it got. Just grow old, get fat, and accept that as the way life is.

You can have that if you want, but it doesn't have to be that way. You are the master of your own fate, no matter your age. If you refuse to accept age as an excuse for mediocrity, you won't be mediocre.

Okay, enough preaching. Let's get back to training.

Volume and Intensity

Regardless of your ability or experience, there are only three workout variables that can be changed in training: duration, frequency, and intensity.

- Duration is how long a given workout is and usually is measured in time.
- Frequency has to with how often the workouts are done. Some athletes work out three times a week and others every day.
- Intensity is a measure of how hard the workout is. It's determined by a rating of perceived exertion, heart rate, pace (or speed), or power.

That's it. Whether you are a former Olympian or brand-new to the sport, those are the only things you can change in your training to produce fitness.

The combination of duration and frequency is called volume. It's always expressed in hours or miles (or kilometers) for a period of time, usually a week. For example, if you work out for an hour a day for an entire week, your volume that week is seven hours.

Introducing volume reduces the training variables to two: volume and intensity. Of these, sport science has been telling us for two decades that the one with the greater impact on performance in *advanced* athletes is intensity.[2] My experience from coaching hundreds of athletes of varying abilities over 30-plus years agrees. But my experience also tells me that for some athletes, a very high volume done at a moderate intensity can sometimes make up for a lack of high-intensity training, especially when the goal event will be raced at a low to moderate intensity, such as a marathon or Ironman triathlon. I've seen some athletes who thrived and performed at a very high level in such events despite the absence of anything in their training we'd call "speed work."

But given the possibility of doing either, I'd prefer to see a mix of an individually reasonable amount of moderate-effort volume along with some high-intensity training. Doing primarily one or the other, I've found, too often ends in injury or a mental breakdown caused by the tedious training.

Could it be that athletes in one sport slow down more than those in another as they get older? And might age-related performance in some sports change more than in others based on the mix of volume and intensity? For example, could high-intensity training be less effective than high volume for older runners but the other way around for older cyclists? There's not much available in the scientific literature on this topic. I know of only one study that's tried to answer these questions, and it produced somewhat open-ended and provocative conclusions.[3]

A cross-sectional study from the University of Bourgogne in France looked at which sport experienced the greatest rates of decline in performance with aging—swimming, cycling, or running. Of course the researchers looked at triathletes to find the answer because they are proficient in all three. In this study, the individual swim, bike, and run times of the top 10 males in each 5-year age group from 20 to 70 were examined at the Triathlon World Championships in 2006 and 2007 for the Olympic distances (swim 1,500 m, bike 40 km, run 10 km) and the Ironman distances (swim 4 km, bike 112 miles, run 26.2 miles). Cycling showed less decline in performance with aging than did running or swimming. And, interestingly, the rate of decline of the categories beyond age 50 for cycling and running was significantly greater for the Ironman athletes. In other words, the older triathletes who raced at the *shorter* distance experienced less decline in performance than those doing the *longer* distance.

This last finding is interesting. Why might that happen? Why would older Ironman athletes get slower at a greater rate as they aged than would their age-related counterparts at the shorter Olympic distance? Of course, the researchers compared the swim, bike, and run split times of, let's say, 50- to 55-year-olds with those of 30- to 35-year-olds at the same distance and then compared the rates of decline for the corresponding Olympic and Ironman age groups. After doing this, the scientists found that the Olympic-distance triathletes slowed down less than their equivalent age peers in the Ironman. They also found that as the athletes got older, they slowed down less in cycling than they did in running. Swimming had a similar and steady decline by age group regardless of the race distance.

Here's my take on this. The primary determiner of performance in short-course racing (events that take about 2 hours to complete) is intensity. In their training, these athletes are likely to do very fast-paced intervals to boost performance. For long-course events (those taking more than 4 hours to finish), the primary determiner of performance is duration, which also means high volume. Long-course athletes are likely to do long, steady workouts at a low intensity. If that's true, and I believe it is, then it seems to point the finger of blame for loss of performance with age at training intensity, not volume. If you train slower, albeit longer, you are likely to lose performance at a greater rate per decade than if you train fast, perhaps with fewer miles.

> **IF YOU TRAIN SLOWER, you are likely to lose performance at a greater rate per decade than if you train fast.**

This brings us back to the big three—the primary determiners of performance decline with age according to sport science. To refresh your memory, these are declining aerobic capacity, increasing body fat, and loss of muscle mass. Let's compare those with the results of the French study of triathletes just described in terms of what apparently had the greatest impact on their performances. As explained in Chapter 3, of the physiological markers of fitness—aerobic capacity, lactate threshold, and economy—aerobic capacity is probably the greater determiner of performance as we age. If that's true, then maintaining or improving aerobic capacity is the best way to get faster (or remain fast) as we get older. The most effective way to improve or maintain aerobic capacity is by doing high-intensity workouts. That, again, supports the research described in previous chapters about how to prevent substantial losses of fitness over the years. Train vigorously with high intensity and you'll stave off a high rate of decline in performance as you age.

This doesn't mean that training volume is of little consequence. In the French study, the Ironman triathletes slowed down less on the bike as they got older compared with both the swim and the run.[4] This may well be because cycling places little stress on muscles, tendons, and joints and can therefore be tolerated for very long periods. It's not unusual for an aging Ironman triathlete to do 5- and 6-hour rides with 10 or more hours per week in the saddle while swimming for about 4 hours and running for 6. More bike time, more bike fitness. So volume apparently has something to do with performance as well.

If you train only a couple of hours weekly, even if they are very intense, it is unlikely that you will approach your potential or be competitive as you get older, especially in traditional endurance events. The best endurance athletes in the world almost always train with intensity *and* with high volume. "High," of course, is a relative term. For a 20-something pro cyclist, high may mean 30 or more hours a week in the saddle. For a competitive 50-year-old age-group marathon runner, 8 hours per week may be high. The same serious runner training for 5K races may run 5 hours a week, and that could be considered high.

So just put in high-volume weeks with a few days of intervals thrown in. No problem, huh?

Well, let's get real. While there certainly are a few athletes who at age 50 (and 60 and even 70) are still putting in very high volume (I know a few of them, and they are certainly remarkable athletes), most of us on the high side of 50 either can't fit high-volume training into our busy lives, or we honestly know that our bodies simply won't handle it. The solution is to find the "Goldilocks volume"—not too high, not too low, but just right. That means just right *for you* given your A-priority race schedule, your available training time, your resistance to injury and illness, and your seasonal training environment. Once you've found this number (it may change throughout the year based on periodization, which we will cover in Chapter 6), stick with it while focusing on intensity. If you make a mistake, make it on the side of too little volume.

Intensity can be sort of tricky, too. The training intensity of an Ironman athlete is significantly different from that of a sprint-distance triathlete. The average training pace of a marathoner is considerably slower than that of a 10K runner. Athletes must train at intensities that are specific to the event for which they are training. Long-distance athletes, such as Ironman triathletes and marathon runners, should not train fast. Or should they? The key is periodization. Again, we'll look for answers to this dilemma in Chapter 6.

High-Intensity Training

Research tells us that the performance decline we typically experience with aging has a lot to do with how active we are while growing older. For example, a paper released in 2000 examined the combined effects of age and activity level over time.[5] The researchers reviewed 242 studies comparing aging and VO_2max involving 13,828 male subjects. Each of the subjects was assigned to one of three groups based on how active they were: sedentary, moderately active exerciser, or endurance-trained runner. Aerobic capacity was highest in the runners and lowest in the sedentary group. No surprises there. The aerobic capacity changes per decade of life were sedentary, 8.7 percent; active, 7.3 percent; runners, 6.8 percent. What this means is if at age 30 a man had a VO_2max of 60 and then for the next 30 years didn't exercise and lived a "normal" (sedentary) life, he could expect his aerobic capacity at age 60 to be around 46. If he was moderately active, it would be about 48. And if he trained as an endurance runner, it would be in the neighborhood of 49. Those are not significant numeric changes. But for normal folks who generally see VO_2max declines of 10 percent and greater for a 10-year period, these numbers are really high.

But regardless of the actual size of the change, here's the main message: The study further reported that the subjects who were endurance-trained runners significantly decreased their volume (miles run per week) and training intensity as they got older. That's a common practice with aging athletes. So maybe it's not simply working out that maintains aerobic capacity and therefore, in part, race performances; instead, it is how much training you do and how intensely you do it.

Yes, I realize that I am repeating the same message. It's a critical lesson for getting faster regardless of your age.

Here's another. Do you remember Michael Pollock's longitudinal study in Chapter 1?[6] It was a watershed study in understanding performance and age, so let's quickly refresh your memory.

In 1987, Dr. Pollock and his colleagues at the Mt. Sinai Medical Center in Milwaukee, Wisconsin, reported an astonishing finding that lent further credibility to the idea that very strenuous exercise was an aerobic capacity preserver. Well-trained, competitive endurance runners with an average initial age of 52 were able to totally maintain VO_2max values over a 10-year period.

In the full group of 24 athletes, VO_2max went into a tailspin, with an average 9 percent decline during the 10 years of the study. However, Pollock discovered that 11 of the 24 had continued to train vigorously and were still competitive a decade after the initial testing. When he categorized the results, he found that the more active athletes had absolutely maintained their average VO_2max at a steady 53 ml/kg/min (10 years earlier it had been 54) despite being now in their early 60s. The less active subjects had seen their VO_2max values plummet by 12 percent. In Pollock's paper, "more active" meant that athletes continued to do high-intensity workouts while maintaining their volume.

Just like Pollock's study, other research on aging in experienced endurance athletes generally supports the notion that in order to reduce the decline in aerobic capacity with advancing age, training must be intense.

That typically means training anaerobically—at or above the lactate threshold. For experienced endurance athletes, an exercise regimen based solely on LSD will do little to improve or even maintain your aerobic fitness status over the years.[7]

Of course, you may not be able to improve it, especially if you've been training intensely for many years. Even with such focused training, there is still the age-related performance decay that research has repeatedly shown us is inevitable. As explained earlier, your history of exercise type and consistency along with your current age have a lot to do with how great your gains may be in the future. If your training has been inconsistent and you are now in your 50s, you're probably more physiologically capable of significantly reversing the downward performance spiral through training than if you have been training consistently or are in your 70s.

That doesn't mean a 70-year-old can't make performance gains after a few years of slacking off. It's just somewhat harder to accomplish due to physiological changes that occur with advancing age, such as reduced hormone production. Hormones have a lot to do with the response to training, fat accumulation, and muscle loss. We'll take a deeper look at this in the next chapter.

There is also the matter of genetics. Some people apparently chose the right parents. They are endowed with a great capacity for hard workouts with little risk of breakdown. They can do high-intensity training and experience a quick and positive response. Others of the same age can do the same workouts over the same time and see little or no performance change. Unfortunately, life isn't always fair.

There's little doubt that intense training is risky. As workouts become more challenging, the chances of injury, illness, and overtraining increase. Intense training needs to be modulated in regard to your current level of fitness and personal age-related limits. Those limits may have become

High-Intensity Training and the Aging Athlete

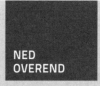

NED
OVEREND

I turned 59 in 2014, and I have maintained a high level of fitness since I first began endurance racing in the late 1970s. Training with an emphasis on high-intensity intervals has been my preferred method of preparing for events throughout my career, which includes racing mountain bikes, road bikes, cyclocross, and XTERRA triathlon. I made a few forays into long-distance events such as the Leadville 100 mountain bike race and the Ironman triathlon, but my preference is racing for 1 to 4 hours.

I embrace a higher-intensity/lower-volume regimen partly because I love to suffer but also because of the race results I've achieved with this philosophy. I have a short attention span for training rides. I like the excitement of pushing the pace both on the climbs and descents as opposed to riding at a slower pace for a longer ride. A long ride for me is about 3 hours, and I rarely do more than one a week.

Early in my career, I noticed that I was able to compete with and often beat riders who trained at much higher volumes, sometimes putting in 20 to 30 percent higher volumes than I did. I'm not saying that my peers should have been training differently, just that I could compete at the highest level while practicing my preferred method of relatively low volume. Racing with a high fitness level while training the way I prefer is a big motivator and the primary reason I have had longevity in endurance sports. As I get older, I need more time to recover, especially from longer rides. This need for recovery time combined with less time to train has made me emphasize intensity over volume even more.

Several studies have shown that although we all lose a certain percentage of our VO_2max over time, maintaining a schedule of high-intensity training significantly cuts the rate of decline in VO_2max .   »

Continued

The two key factors that make training with high intensity possible and beneficial for the aging athlete are proper recovery and the motivation needed to push yourself. Here's how I manage these at age 59.

I've learned that by reducing volume, I'm more rested for high-intensity sessions, and by being rested, I can push myself harder during the intervals. Getting quality recovery by including massage, stretching, hydration, nutrition, and sleep enables me to build momentum in my fitness program.

For motivation, I find that a mix of joining group workouts and using the website Strava (http://www.strava.com) is effective in helping me to push my intensity to high levels. Whether it's our local Durango, Colorado, Tuesday-night "world championships" or the Specialized Bicycles lunch ride, whenever I ride in a group training situation, I'm motivated to push myself. I know a lot of riders avoid these group rides because their egos get hurt if they get dropped, but the best way to get better at group rides is to do them. Learn when to pull and when to sit in, and determine what strategy you need to stay on as long as possible. Suffering is less noticeable in a group dynamic; you don't have as much focus on the »

magnified by the absence of high-intensity training in recent years. If that's the case, you need to be extraconservative with training changes as you ease into what I'm going to propose.

If high-intensity training is something you haven't done for a long time or have never done, you must consider several things: the type of hard workouts, the frequency of hard workouts, your short-term recovery from hard workouts, and your nutrition relative to hard workouts. I'll cover these points in Chapters 6, 7, and 8. But for now, let's look at high-intensity training for aerobic capacity.

pain of the effort when you are making sure that you hang on to the wheel in front of you. Jumping across gaps or working with other riders to maintain a gap becomes a type of shared group pain, and I find it helps me push harder than when I train alone.

Strava plays a big role in my specific high-intensity intervals. I have always pushed myself on certain segments in my training rides. If I am training for a power race, I do intervals on the flats and rollers. If there is race coming up with long climbs, I simulate that in my training. Now that Strava has become popular, course segments have start and finish lines, and I'm racing not only my own PR but also that of every other Strava. With the help of the Strava segments, I've learned how to pace myself, where to go hard, and where to conserve effort in order to reduce my time. It's a great motivational tool.

I think the major reason I've been a successful endurance racer is that I've determined the right intensity-recovery ratio for me. It's not static—it changes with my personal stress level, altitude, age, illness, injury, and more. I'm careful not to deceive myself by greedily overtraining because going hard has no value without proper recovery.

Guidelines for High-Intensity Training

The most effective and efficient use of your time and energy to increase training intensity is to do some type of interval training.[8]

Important point: When you perform intervals, the absolute intensity, the duration of the repetitions, the number of repetitions, and the duration of recovery between intervals must be only slightly more challenging than your estimated current capacity for physical stress.

What that means is that you must know or be able to sense your physical limits and not exceed them. It's best to take a conservative approach to intervals if it's been a while since you last did such a workout. Don't try to get in shape in just a handful of these sessions. Too much, too soon will nearly always result in a breakdown of some sort, such as injury. Take a long-term approach—as in several weeks—to safely produce the results you want.

Because an interval session can be quite stressful, it should be preceded by a gradually progressive warm-up. This approach has also been shown to improve workout performance.[9] Stop the workout when a reasonable workout goal is attained, when it is apparent that high-end performance is declining, or when the effort feels unusually high for the output (pace, speed, power). My advice to the athletes I've coached for the past 30-some years has always been the same: Stop when you know you can do only one more interval. The last interval is the one to be most wary of, so simply don't do it.

Note that I am not going to describe specific interval workouts for each individual endurance sport. I am going to assume that as a lifelong athlete, you are familiar with interval training and that you either have a record of or remember the interval workouts for your sport that have worked for you in the past. If this is not the case, you will need to research the proper interval training for your sport.

I am also not going to prescribe specific methodology for measuring intensity. Again, I am going to assume that your years in your sport have given you a strong foundation in monitoring the intensity of your workouts. You can use a rating of perceived exertion (RPE), heart rate, lactate threshold heart rate, or functional threshold power if you are using a power meter and are familiar with that measurement. Go with whatever you are comfortable using and whatever is most repeatable for you.

I recommend that you keep track of your heart rate even if you do not use it to measure intensity. Heart rate is a useful component in determining the state of your fitness and the rate at which you are improving it, as you will see below.

If you have been diagnosed with coronary heart disease, have concerns about your heart health, or are taking statins or other medications that alter heart rate, then you should consult your doctor before starting an interval training program. Fortunately, the risk of heart attack among otherwise apparently healthy athletes as they age is quite low.[10]

If you've previously done intervals throughout your sport career but have had a gap in recent years, then you know how to get started again. Just be conservative (as I mentioned before) with the progression of this workout. If LSD training has been your only training method, you may need some guidelines for getting started with interval training. Here is what I suggest for the first few sessions for someone who has not done interval training recently.

Step 1. *Warm up 10–30 minutes gradually, ratcheting intensity up to a moderate effort.* It's common for older athletes to need more warm-up time than young athletes. Warm-up may also vary by sport. For example, it is typically longer for cycling than for running. Swimming generally falls between these two.

Step 2. *Do 3 × 3-minute intervals with each interval at or slightly below lactate (anaerobic) threshold and 1 minute of light recovery between them.* As I mentioned before, the gauge of intensity for an interval workout such as this may be based on heart rate, pace, speed, power, or perceived exertion. Some of these measurements are better than others, depending on the sport (see Appendix C). Heart rate–based intensity is perhaps the worst way to gauge how hard to work with intervals, especially short ones of a few minutes or less, as heart rate rises slowly during each interval. It may take several minutes to achieve lactate threshold, during which time you are left guessing how hard to work. Most athletes err on the side of starting intervals too fast to force heart rate up quickly, and then they slow down later as the goal heart rate is finally achieved. This is just the opposite of what should be done; instead, you want to finish each interval with a slightly higher intensity than when you started.

Step 3. *Cool down with several minutes of easy exercise.* As with the warm-up, the duration of the cooldown depends on the sport, with cycling typically long and running relatively short.

At first you should most likely do only one such interval workout in a seven-day period. Over time, however, you can increase the number of weekly sessions to two if you have the stamina and time. It's not common for senior athletes to be capable of doing more than two of these in a week. I've coached some who could, but they are rare and more likely in their 50s than their 70s.

An indicator of improving fitness is that the speed or power of your intervals increases relative to your heart rate (this is where keeping track of your heart rate during interval training comes in, as mentioned before). That's always a sure sign of improving aerobic fitness. To determine this, divide the *combined* average speed (run, swim, Nordic ski) or normalized power (bike or row) for all of the intervals by their *combined* average heart rate (see my book *The Power Meter Handbook* for details on this). The increase in this ratio is the indicator that your aerobic fitness is improving. TrainingPeaks (www.trainingpeaks.com) calls this ratio the "efficiency factor" (EF).

For example, let's say you did 3 × 3-minute intervals running at just below lactate threshold, and the combined average pace of the intervals was

7:15 per mile. To convert pace to speed, divide 60 by 7.25, and you'll find that the speed of the intervals was 8.3 mph. That's a speed of 243 yards per minute (8.3 × 1,760 yards in a mile divided by 60, the number of minutes in an hour). Yards and minutes are easier to work with than miles and hours for our purpose. And let's say the combined average heart rate of all of the intervals was 150. That means your EF for that workout was 1.62 (243 ÷ 150 = 1.62). As that number increases, your aerobic fitness is also improving.

Now, if you don't have a pacing or power device, or even a heart rate monitor—or if using those tools seems like too much math and measurement—we can simplify the decision regarding when to bump your intervals up. If you are familiar with the RPE method mentioned earlier, you probably know it isn't nearly as accurate as power meters, pacing devices, and heart rate monitors, but it'll do in a pinch. Simply do the intervals at the same *perceived effort* as usual and make a conscious determination during the intervals whether you seem to be going faster than the last time you did them. If you are on a measured course, you can time your intervals. This effort will never be "easy." But if you do the intervals at roughly the same effort each time, over time you will go faster as fitness improves. The RPE method is best on a measured course using a stopwatch. Old school, but it still works.

When you are going faster at the same level of effort, it's time to make some changes. As the EF for your interval sessions rises (meaning you get faster at the same effort), you will need to increase the number of intervals. As these longer interval workouts become more tolerable with a rising EF, begin to gradually increase the duration of the individual intervals. The recovery time between them should be about one-third of the preceding interval time. For example, after a 3-minute interval, recover for 1 minute. When you can manage about 20 minutes of total combined interval time in a single workout (such as 4 intervals of 5 minutes each at lactate threshold with 1 minute 40 seconds of recovery between them), then you are ready to move on to more intense intervals.

The next stage in the progression for those just getting back into high-intensity training is to move up to aerobic-capacity intervals. To do this, start with 5 to 10 intervals of 30 to 60 seconds each with recoveries between them *of the same duration*, for a total of 5 minutes of intervals in a single session (e.g., 10 × 30 seconds or 5 × 60 seconds). This time, however, do them *above* the lactate threshold. As a memory refresher: Lactate threshold is the intensity at which you first begin to experience labored breathing. You should feel as if you are working quite hard on these aerobic-capacity intervals, but they aren't *quite* an all-out effort.

Aerobic-capacity speed or power is the highest average speed or power you can sustain for about 5 minutes. If you really want to know what that number is for you right now (it varies with changes in fitness), do an all-out 5-minute time trial on your own to find your average speed or power for that duration. Or you could have a VO_2max test done in a university lab, medical clinic, health club, or sporting goods store or by a coach. If you go the test route, be sure to ask the technician what your top-end or VO_2max speed or power was.

Rather than doing a time trial or lab test, you can get a rough estimate of your VO_2max output by multiplying your speed or power at lactate threshold (perhaps found in the round of intervals described above) by 1.05 and 1.2. That will give you a range to shoot for on each of these aerobic-capacity intervals. Start at the low end of this range, and over time gradually increase the intensity to the upper end.

In Chapters 5 and 6, we'll get into the details of doing the advanced aerobic-capacity interval workout.

If you prefer to be somewhat less structured in your training, do these initial VO_2max intervals as "fartlek." That's a Swedish term for "speed play" that has been commonly used by athletes, especially runners, for the past 70 years to mean "unstructured intervals." To do such a workout, start with a warm-up. Then go fast when you feel like it, go slow when you feel like it, and complete as many of these fast segments as you feel like doing. As explained earlier, you still must pay attention to how you feel throughout the workout, being cautious not to do so many fast segments that you can't fully recover within three days.

YOU CAN MAKE short-term improvements that produce immediate results while also greatly slowing the long-term losses.

After a few weeks, and once you are fully adapted to high-intensity training, your aerobic capacity should be increasing. You can measure that as before with the 5-minute time trial, or you can undergo a technician-administered test. You may also simply discover that you're going faster in your workouts for the same effort. Depending on your fitness at the start of this program, your rate of workout progression, the number of such sessions completed, and your age, it would not be unusual to see a 5 percent improvement in VO_2max in about eight weeks. And by continuing such training in future years, your rate of loss of aerobic capacity should be no greater than about 5 percent *per decade*.

What if your personal limiter isn't aerobic capacity but rather lactate threshold? Just because nearly all of the research has found VO_2max to be the aging athlete's primary limiter, it doesn't necessarily mean it's that way for *all* serious senior athletes.

First let me say that this situation is rare. Nevertheless, it would likely be the case if your known VO_2max or 5-minute time trial speed has declined by less than about 5 percent per decade, or around half a percentage point in a year. If this describes your recent experience, then you may benefit from devoting a good portion of your training to sub-lactate-threshold sessions, as described earlier. That could mean fewer aerobic-capacity interval sessions. Note, however, that some research has found that doing aerobic-capacity intervals is also an effective way to boost lactate threshold.[11] So both types of intervals may improve your fitness even if your aerobic capacity is stable.

Let's move on to another form of high-intensity training that addresses one of the other big three limiters for senior athletes: the loss of muscle mass with aging.

Strength Training

Although many (maybe most) endurance athletes believe their hearts should be the central focus of training for high performance, the loss of fitness with aging largely depends on muscle. The heart is only a pump that responds to the needs of the muscles by speeding up or slowing down its rhythm to meet the muscles' demands. If you want to be highly fit, focus first and primarily on your sport-specific muscles.

Muscle training does *not* mean trying to develop big, bulging muscles. That is unlikely to produce any endurance benefit and is more likely to harm performance. What you really need is lots of strong, aerobically active muscle, especially when it comes to the muscles that are the primary movers in your sport. For a runner and a cyclist, those muscles are mostly found in the legs. But they aren't necessarily the same muscles; nor do they operate in the same way for both of these leg-powered sports. Similarly, for a swimmer, rower, or paddler, the muscles that drive the arms are critical to performance, but training in one of these arm-dominant sports does not ensure success in the others.

Aerobically active muscles are those that have an abundance of endurance qualities. These are the slow-twitch muscles, the ones that aren't very powerful but can repeat their contractions many times before fatiguing. They are also called "type I" fibers and are quite common in the sport-specific muscles of endurance athletes. In contrast, fast-twitch muscles are powerful but fatigue quite rapidly. These "type II" muscle fibers are abundant in power athletes such as sprinters. There are several subtypes within these two divisions, which are not yet fully understood by science. There is reason to believe that some type II subtypes are capable of taking on the slow-twitch qualities of type I.[12] And the opposite may be true as well.[13]

Of course, the greater concern for us as endurance athletes is the possible conversion of type I to type II, marking a loss of endurance muscle. Fortunately, that is highly unlikely to happen. The more common shift is the other way around. Some type II fast-twitch muscles can take on the endurance characteristics of our type I buddies. That would increase your endurance and also your power, as even in such a conversion, not all of the power qualities of the type II fibers are likely to be lost. In this case, conversion would be beneficial. You'd have both slightly more power and more endurance.

Unfortunately, if you focus only on LSD training, your type II fibers could possibly decrease in number and not become slow twitch–like. That's just another appearance by our old friend *use it or lose it*. How can you prevent this from happening? One way is through high-intensity, sport-specific training—aerobic-capacity intervals—as described earlier. Another way is through strength training, what athletes typically call lifting weights.

As a senior athlete, can you still increase your strength? The answer is a definite yes. Sedentary people of all ages, including in their 80s, have successfully improved muscle strength with weight lifting.[14] As with all high-intensity training, however, the risk of injury when lifting weights is fairly high. Just as with aerobic-capacity intervals, if you have not done resistance training for some time, you may well injure a joint or even your low back. Care must be taken to progress from light to heavy loads gradually over several weeks. (For details, see Chapter 6 and Appendix A.)

The best time to start a strength training program is early in your Base period. That's 20 or more weeks prior to your first A-priority race. To complete such a program—from starting with 20 reps to eventually finishing several sessions of about 3 to 9 reps—will take several weeks. Once you've completed this program, move into a strength maintenance program for the remainder of the buildup to the first race of the season. In a maintenance program, you do only 2 sets of each exercise in a session, and you do only 1 session per week. One set is moderately heavy (10 to 15 reps) and is done as a warm-up; the second is heavy (3 to 9 reps). These are very brief workouts. If you return to base training following the first race, also return to an earlier phase of strength training. For some, that may mean doing a few sessions of 3 sets of 3 to 9 reps with heavy loads. (All of this is explained in greater detail in Chapter 6.)

Lifting weights can significantly improve your race performances if you haven't trained that way before.[15] Essentially, when you train with heavy loads for several weeks, you develop younger muscles, which are capable of greater endurance performance.[16] If you stop lifting weights for several weeks before your first race, you are likely to experience a loss of strength and muscle. This is more likely for the oldest age groups, such as 70 and higher, than for 50-year-olds.

The High-Performance Senior Athlete

If it's been years since you've done high-intensity workouts that involve aerobic-capacity intervals and strength training, there is little doubt that you will see a significant improvement in training and performance by starting such a program. You will also see a change in how fast you age—

meaning how slowly your aerobic capacity and muscle are lost in the coming years. The average intensity of your training will increase. Intensity, not duration, is the key to high performance in experienced athletes.

The third key to improving performance and decreasing fitness losses over time is maintaining a lean body. That's at least as important as aerobic-capacity training and weight lifting. We'll get into that topic in Chapter 8.

When you are training with high intensity, you must be cautious with the progression both of the aerobic-capacity intervals and heavy loads at the gym. The risk of injury is quite high. Never train through discomfort or pain when a muscle, tendon, or joint is complaining about what you are doing to it that day. Always stop as soon as this happens. Believing the discomfort or pain will go away if you continue is always the wrong approach. You risk losing several days, weeks, or even months of training by pushing on. Stop and take care of the soreness. This may involve seeking medical help.

It's a good idea to include lactate-threshold interval training in your program along with aerobic-capacity intervals. Even for the athlete who can manage multiple high-intensity sessions in a week, long, steady intervals done at or slightly below lactate threshold are quite effective for maintaining or even improving performance. In fact, if you are unable to do aerobic-capacity intervals for any reason, lactate-threshold training is the way to go.

Fitting aerobic-capacity intervals, lactate-threshold training, and strength training into a week can be quite a challenge for many aging athletes. In Chapter 6, I'll propose a novel way that you might resolve this conundrum.

To be sure, even with high-intensity training, it's not possible to *completely* stop the decline in aerobic capacity and muscle mass over the course of several years. But you can make short-term improvements that produce immediate performance results while also greatly slowing the long-term losses. As you read in Chapter 1, if you continue down the road of doing only LSD training, your losses are likely to be in the range of 1 percent per year or greater. High-intensity training has been shown to cut that in half. And that's where you want to be.

TRAINING BASICS

The afternoon knows what the morning never suspected.

—ROBERT FROST

Training is stressful. It's meant to be. If it wasn't, there would be no fitness. To understand the principles of training stress, we have to go back to the 1930s, when a young medical student at the University of Prague by the name of Hans Selye came up with an idea he called "General Adaptation Syndrome" (GAS).[1] Later, in his medical practice and as a college professor in endocrinology at the University of Montreal, he continued to refine this concept. Today his ideas of how stress affects us are still studied and have been applied to training for endurance sports.

Selye's GAS theory explains how animals—including athletes—adapt and grow stronger or weaker as a result of stress. According to his theory, there are two types of stress: distress and eustress.[2] *Distress* is what we normally think of when the word "stress" is used. That's the "bad" stress, the type that detracts from our health and well-being and often leads to illness, anxiety, withdrawal, and depression. This sounds like overtraining, doesn't it? But there is also "good" stress. That's *eustress*. This is the type of stress that keeps you healthy and produces fitness. Its common symptoms are feelings of vigor, well-being, and satisfaction. Without eustress, there would be no reason to exercise. You would never become stronger or race faster. Training would be meaningless.

Moderation and Consistency

Based on Selye's concepts, sports scientists have developed a theory of how the human body adapts to training. It's called "supercompensation."[3] Figure 5.1 illustrates their theory of how we gain fitness as a result of training eustress. Here you can see that as hard training progresses, fitness is gradually lost. That's because fatigue is accumulating. Over several days of challenging workouts, even with a few easy recovery workouts sprinkled in here and there, the body is slowly breaking down. In sport science, this is called "catabolism." Supercompensation occurs when the body is finally allowed a few days of decreased training for rest and recovery. At that point, the athlete gains an increase in fitness as the body is restructured. This process is "anabolism" (rebuilding) kicking in to restructure the organs and tissues so that they are capable of handling more stress in the future. The athlete can now train at a *slightly* greater workload—more volume or more intensity or both—in the next block of training. As you already know from your years of training, this pattern is repeated over and over throughout the season, resulting in much-improved fitness over time.

The obvious conclusion we can draw from this pattern is that hard training only creates the potential for fitness. True fitness isn't realized until the athlete is allowed to rest and recover by reducing the training load for a few days.

FIGURE 5.1. **Supercompensation occurs between training blocks**

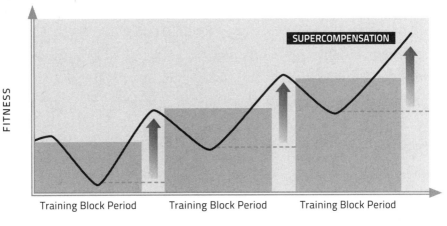

Without frequent periods of reduced training, there is no supercompensation and no increase in fitness. Were you to omit the rest and recovery breaks, the downward-sloping lines of Figure 5.1 would simply continue to plummet. Training would become *distress*. In sport, we call this "overtraining." The cause of overtraining is always too little rest and recovery accompanied by too much volume or too much intensity (or both). While there is no research on this, there is reason to believe that older athletes may become overtrained with a smaller training load over a shorter period of time than younger athletes, which indicates that older athletes need to monitor their training load carefully. The tools in this chapter will help you do so.

I've known athletes who were overtrained. It isn't pretty. It takes huge motivation to produce this sad condition because the body does everything it can to stop us from continuing to train without rest. For some, however, training may continue due to their addiction to the opiumlike chemicals the body releases during exercise—dopamine and endorphins.[4]

Athletes who crave the boost they get from the release of these neu-rotransmitters and proteins simply can't stop.

Fortunately, the body has ways of forestalling the effects of overtrain-ing.[5] Fatigue is its best preventive tool. Exhaustion steadily increases with overtraining and becomes so great that getting out of bed in the morning is difficult. General malaise gradually develops and continues throughout the day, every day. Relentlessly. The body gradually introduces more ways of stopping the distress. Motivation to do anything physical reaches a low point. Appetite decreases, and body weight is lost. Muscular soreness may develop. Upper respiratory illnesses are common. The athlete becomes moody and is often grumpy. The list of symptoms goes on and on. The distress simply becomes overwhelming. And yet some athletes are so highly motivated or addicted that they press ahead.

Clearly, it takes extreme dedication to one's sport to fall victim to over-training. Most athletes are simply incapable of continuing beyond the onset of extreme fatigue. It's too difficult for most of us to train through such distress. The mind may be willing, but the body is incapable.

How should an athlete distinguish between the signs of healthy train-ing fatigue and the symptoms of overtraining? Fatigue is a common marker of training and is normal and necessary to produce the potential for fitness. The difference is that this fatigue disappears with a few days of reduced training. Such fatigue is a symptom of eustress. The athlete's con-dition is now called "overreaching." This kind of fatigue is a common sign that your training will produce supercompensation. It's also a warning that should you continue to increase the workload without frequent rest and recovery breaks, overtraining is imminent.

The key to avoiding the danger of overtraining is periodization.[6] Peri-odization is nothing more than creating a careful plan for your training that allows you to build in periods of intense exercise that cause fatigue, balanced by periods of recovery that encourage the body to rebuild and grow stronger. We'll explore that topic with a unique solution to the problem in Chapter 6. And in Chapter 7 we'll study the intricacies of recovery.

A second tool to monitor your training load and avoid overtraining is to regularly test your degree of fitness and to measure your progress toward your training and racing goals. We'll cover the different ways to monitor your fitness later in this chapter.

PERIODIZATION is the key to avoiding the danger of overtraining.

For now, I want to emphasize that some fatigue is okay and normal, but if you ever experience extreme fatigue that doesn't go away with a few days of rest and recovery, and that feeling is accompanied by any of the other signs of overtraining mentioned earlier, do not assume you are merely suffering from a temporary and easily corrected condition akin to a head cold. Overtraining can be career-ending.

There are also separate health issues to be aware of. The overtraining symptoms described above don't automatically mean that you're overtrained—you could be dealing with something worse in the form of a disease. If the signs of overtraining appear, make an appointment to see your doctor immediately. There are many ailments that present with symptoms similar to those of overtraining, such as mononucleosis and Lyme disease. If testing for these diseases and others comes back with negative results, you may then assume that you're dealing with overtraining. If that's the case, you will need a lot of rest, which in turn unfortunately means a still greater loss of fitness. This is not something to take lightly. It may take weeks or even months of greatly reduced exercise before you begin to bounce back.

The take-home message is that you must always respect fatigue if you are to gain fitness. To race fast after 50, make it your goal to train consistently and moderately with adequate rest and recovery. In Chapter 4 we saw the logic of *conservatively* increasing high-intensity training. Increase your aerobic-capacity intervals gradually in regard to interval duration and total high-intensity time in a single workout. The rate at which you ramp up the training loads when lifting weights must also be conservative. Don't force your body to become fit; gently persuade it. Remember: eustress, not distress.

If there is one thing you have undoubtedly learned in your 50-plus years on this planet, it's that life is not a sprint; it's a marathon. Sprinting in a marathon is a sure way to crash and burn. In much the same way, your aerobic capacity and muscular strength simply cannot increase exponentially by tomorrow. Be patient with your body. Always take a long-term, gradual, and conservative approach to high-intensity training. Allow several months, perhaps an entire season, to become faster by training moderately and consistently. It will pay off with deep fitness that stays with you for the long haul.

What can you do to ensure that your training is moderate and therefore consistent? That's what we will delve into in the remainder of this chapter.

Risk and Reward

Every workout has a potential risk and also a possible reward. "Risk" refers not only to overtraining but also to injury, illness, mental burnout, and other breakdowns that may occur because a workout or a closely spaced series of workouts is overly challenging. "Reward" has to do with the fitness and performance benefits that result from training. In your training you should seek to balance these two variables.

You can't have a reward without taking some risk. That's just the way life is. For example, using these same terms, we could be talking about making

FIGURE 5.2. **The risk-reward curves of training**

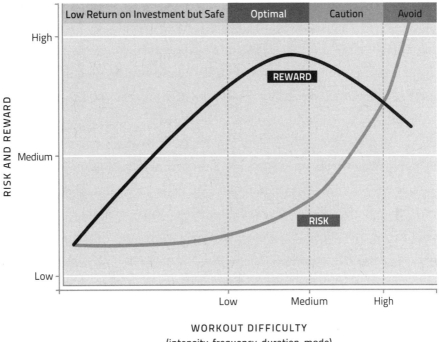

WORKOUT DIFFICULTY
(intensity, frequency, duration, mode)

investment decisions. You could put your hard-earned money into bonds that have low risk. They also tend to have a small reward, and you cannot expect to become rich overnight by investing this way. Low risk almost always means low reward. On the other hand, you could choose to invest in a start-up company that has great promise in a new field of technology that has vast potential. If the company and the new technology succeed, you could multiply your investment a hundredfold. Then again, if the company fails or the technology doesn't pan out, you could lose every cent. High risk means a potentially high reward. It's much the same with training.

Figure 5.2 illustrates the risk–reward curves of training. Your goal should be to put in a lot of training in the "optimal" zone, only a little training in the "caution" zone, and none in the "avoid" zone. The "low return but safe" zone is primarily for recovery sessions, aerobic-threshold development, and maintenance. Unfortunately, this latter part is where most of us who are north of age 50 increasingly spend our training time. To avoid training without improvement, we need to put in time in the "optimal" and "caution" zones, which is where high-intensity training fits in.

How do you determine which zone you are in during a workout? Much depends on variables that include your current level of fitness, your sport experience, how well rested you are, your recent diet, and the psychological stress in your life. The proper workload for any workout is based largely on what you know about yourself. As an experienced athlete, you can pair your lifelong response to training with your knowledge of intensity levels, using whichever method you have employed to monitor intensity throughout your athletic career. But if in doubt about how long or hard a high-intensity session should be, err on the low side. As you learn more about such training and how your body responds to it, your workouts will become more refined and will more closely match your needs.

Risk

The riskiest training most commonly involves the possibility of overuse injuries. Running is perhaps the riskiest endurance sport due primarily to the orthopedic stress, or pounding, associated with it. In fact, runners without a history of injuries are rare. Soft but firm running surfaces, such as trails, grass, and dirt, moderate some of the risk of running. But running is inherently risky due to its eccentric muscle contractions, wherein a muscle lengthens as it is trying to shorten. This sounds impossible, but visualize a reverse arm curl in which you slowly lower a heavy weight. As the weight is lowered, the biceps gets longer at the same time that it is trying to shorten to prevent gravity from making the load fall too fast. The strain on the muscle is tremendous. The runner's calf and quads experi-ence this phenomenon with every step. That's why a runner's legs are so sore after a marathon. Essentially, the muscles are being pulled apart.

Cycling, Nordic skiing, rowing, and swimming, on the other hand, rely primarily on concentric contractions, meaning the muscle only gets shorter as it contracts. Visualize your arm curling a heavy weight from hip height to shoulder height. The strain on the muscle is reduced. It's not being pulled apart, so the risk of injury is lower.

Runners must be extremely cautious with risk in their attempt to reap a reward. Workloads that have a low to moderate risk in other sports may be in the "avoid" zone in running. If you are a runner, you should be espe-cially concerned with training moderation. Should you also have a history of overuse injuries, you must do everything you can to mitigate risk by training with caution and moderation while getting adequate recovery.

Swimming is one of the lowest-risk sports. While overuse injuries cer-tainly occur among swimmers (mostly in the shoulder), the rate of such setbacks is low compared with that of runners. Poor technique and the use of paddles and drag or resistance devices increase the risk for swim-mers, as does rapidly increasing the volume and intensity of training.

Cycling is a similar story, although here the knee is the body part most commonly injured from too much training stress. Risk is increased in cycling first and foremost through poor bike setup. The most common bike setups that are high-risk for the knee have the saddle too low and too far forward. These errors are common for novices, but older athletes can fall into the same mistakes when they make adjustments to compensate for limited mobility in the shoulders and neck. Also raising the risk for cyclists is high-gear pedaling, especially on hills in the seated position. Inadequate gearing, meaning not enough low gears, is often associated with knee soreness and loss of training time due to injury.

Another potentially rewarding activity that carries a high degree of risk for athletes in many sports is plyometrics, especially the kind that includes a lot of landings at the end of downward jumps—jumping over objects or off high platforms, for example. Jumping up from the floor to land on a knee-high box has a much lower risk but also a lower reward. Be cautious with plyometrics, and progress at a quite moderate rate.

Lifting weights is also risky, especially when the loads are high and the reps low. As with intervals, the key to managing the risk is progression—how quickly you increase the loads. The key, as always, is to take a moderate approach when doing reps and adding weight. Stay below the risk curve by doing fewer reps than you think are possible—don't go to "failure" on a set—and be patient about advancing to the next level of training. Be especially cautious with exercises that place great loads on the knees, shoulders, and low back. Injury to these areas is quite common in weight lifters who don't moderate the risk.

Athletes who continually experience breakdowns because they over-invest in high-risk training will never achieve their potential. Likewise, those who do only low-risk workouts will never come close to their potential. Some risk in training is required to reap a reward. You need to control that risk with moderation to be successful. You are the only one who knows what the risk is and what "moderation" means for you. If you are unsure or don't trust yourself to make wise decisions in managing risk, you should hire a coach or trainer. Find someone who is experienced in working with senior athletes in your specific sport.

Reward

That's the risk side of training. How about the rewards? Exactly what positive outcomes can you expect as a result of high-intensity training? In Chapter 4, I described the benefits of increased aerobic capacity from doing

Osteoarthritis and the Aging Athlete

JOHN POST, MD

The *Journal of the American Medical Association* noted recently that "currently, 52.5 million U.S. adults—22.7% of men and women aged 18 years or older—report having arthritis that was diagnosed by a physician" and that 43.2 percent of them said arthritis pain restricts their activities. I am one of them.

I'm a six-time Kona finisher who wouldn't (or couldn't) do the event again if you paid me. In other words, I'm discovering one of the reasons that there are fewer racers in each age group as we age. But on the other side of that coin, yes, I have arthritis, but I won my age group at my last sprint triathlon. Having an age-related condition like arthritis does not mean you need to give up your sport. You may, however, need to make some modifications in how you approach it.

Walt Stack, or "the Amazing Walt Stack," as he was referred to in his hometown of San Francisco, was 73 years of age in 1981, the first year the Ironman was held on the Big Island in Hawaii. Stack was the oldest competitor in the event and was very fond of saying, "Start off slow and taper back." He still holds the record for the Kona course—the record for the longest time, that is, of 26 hours, 20 minutes. So it doesn't look like age or arthritis knocks everyone out.

Not a great deal is known about avoiding the development of arthritis. When we use this term, we're specifically referring to the wear that sometimes occurs to the cartilage that lines our joints. The knee seems to be the most commonly involved area in the sports community, and keeping our weight down has been shown to be the single most important variable under our control. You can't modify your genetics or change the past if you've had trauma to the joint or meniscus surgery, but you certainly don't need to give up hope.

»

Continued

Many find that consistent, knowledgeable joint care by athlete and caregiver together works best. As explained in detail in the book *Triathlon Science*, coedited by Joe Friel and Jim Vance, having an available injury resource team can keep us pain-free, or nearly so, so that we can continue to train and race even with advancing age. We may have to be a little flexible in training or race scheduling, backing off from both when in pain, and we may need to consider crosstraining or pool running. With a little patience and the right treatment, we can still "stay in the game," as they say on TV.

Occasional use of Tylenol or nonsteroidal anti-inflammatories such as ibuprofen and naproxen can go a long way. Even cortisone injections into the joint are permitted by the U.S. Anti-Doping Agency regulations. Given the right circumstances, these drugs can aid the arthritic athlete enormously. In a very few cases, there may be a limited role for arthroscopy to "clean out" the arthritic joint. Should you need a joint replacement, become a race volunteer!

Like many other changes that occur as we age, arthritis may be "just one of those things," but it's not one that needs to put us out of commission. Treat it with a little patience, education, and understanding. Develop a plan, be willing to alter it, possibly redefine your goal, and look at the sport through a glass that is always at least half full.

intervals and greater aerobically active muscle mass as a result of weight lifting. All of those deliver greater performance for athletes. But there's more to expect from high-intensity training that is especially enticing to senior athletes. This enticement has to do with hormones, those chemicals the body produces in the glands that regulate our health and physiology.

As with most aging conditions, we have some degree of control over our hormones. You can somewhat speed up or slow down your body's anabolic hormone production based on your lifestyle and training. The hormones involved include testosterone, human growth hormone, and insulinlike growth factor. When these are released into the body by the glands, they stimulate tissue growth and repair. In fact, without them there would be no improvement in fitness and performance.

Another anabolic hormone underproduced with advancing age is erythropoietin (EPO). That's also the name of a synthetic drug cycling has been dealing with since the early 1990s that was involved with the fall from grace of Lance Armstrong and numerous other athletes. While synthetic EPO is to be avoided, erythropoietin is produced normally by the body and controls red-blood-cell production. Interestingly, it's also associated with memory. And, perhaps more importantly, it is related to your aerobic capacity. Less naturally occurring EPO means fewer red blood cells, resulting in less oxygen being transported to the muscles and therefore a reduced aerobic capacity.

Unfortunately, all anabolic hormone production, including EPO, greatly diminishes with age.[7] This accounts for much of the physiological change that's taking place in our sports performance north of 50. But here's the good news: High-intensity training stimulates anabolic hormone secretion more than does low-intensity, steady-state training.[8] Heavy-load strength training has a similar effect.[9] Following such workouts, hormonal secretion also remains high during the extended recovery period. The results of studies using both older and younger subjects and females as well as males found similar benefits across the board.[10]

Hormone secretion is especially high when you are asleep, the key being the consistency of sleep over time rather than the duration of your snoozing.[11] Just as with the average intensity of your workouts, getting to bed at a regular time appears to be important for natural hormone production. Irregular sleep patterns and a steady diet of only long, slow distance year after year while avoiding the weight room is likely to result in a significant and steady decline in hormonal activity and therefore fitness-related performance. If you're like most older athletes, sleep isn't the problem; training intensity is.

The latter point is why I've been encouraging you to do some of your training near your aerobic capacity with intervals while also lifting heavy weights. Both of these must be done regularly and consistently if you are to reap the hormonal rewards. There is no doubt that such training can be risky, so you must be conservative when starting this sort of training and cautious with increasing the workloads. I can't emphasize enough how critical this is. Always think in terms of moderation as you train in order to minimize risk. Be patient. No injuries. No overtraining.

Measuring Your Progress

For the serious athlete, regardless of age, the key question as the season progresses is: Am I becoming fitter and faster? That question will ultimately be answered when you race, of course, but by then it's too late to do anything about it. What you need is frequent feedback from training about how you are progressing with race preparation. The way to get that feedback is to measure your progress, the more often the better.

Your perceptions of how you feel during workouts have merit. Does today's workout seem easier than usual? Sensing that you are more fit is certainly good feedback. But it's a rather rough estimate involving a recollection of and a comparison with how you felt the last time you did a similar workout. A hard workout that feels a bit easier than the last one is a nice indicator that something positive is happening. However, it isn't precise: "Feel" cannot be relied upon as an accurate measure of fitness.

But measurement usually means numbers, and accurate measurement always involves tools. A carpenter uses a tape measure before sawing. A farmer measures a field's productivity in bushels. A doctor measures body temperature with a thermometer. Without accurate measurement, you are left wondering whether your training plan is working.

The most basic measurement tool that we use in sports is a stopwatch, of course. Endurance athletes have used time to gauge their progress for well over a century. That's still how race performance is measured in most endurance sports. Running is a perfect example. The first official world-record time for the mile on a track was established in 1852, when Charles Westhall from Great Britain was clocked at 4:28.0. The current men's world record of 3:43.13 was set in 1999 by Hicham el Guerrouj of Morocco.[12] How fast you are is nearly always the most important measurement in a race. The challenge in using a stopwatch is controlling for the weather and the course. Wind, ambient temperature, course surface, and topography greatly affect time.

YOUR PERCEPTIONS of how you feel during workouts have merit.

There are other tools you can use in addition to a stopwatch. Most endurance athletes have heart rate monitors. They've been around since the late 1970s and are relatively inexpensive as training tools go. Measuring heart rate tells you the level of your effort—how hard you are working. That's good information and, as I'll show you shortly, can be used to help measure fitness changes. Heart rate alone, however, doesn't tell you anything about performance, even if you know your training zones. The last-place finisher may have exactly the same average heart rate and have been in the same zone as the race winner. All we know is that both worked hard. For an experienced and serious athlete who trains regularly, heart rate doesn't change appreciably, even though fitness may.[13] So knowing *only* your heart rate doesn't tell you anything about your fitness. It needs to be compared with something else to truly be a fitness measurement. Hold that thought, as we'll come back to it shortly.

A more recent tool for athletes in most sports is the speed-and-distance device, more commonly known as a sport GPS and accelerometer. The beauty of such a device is that you don't have to work out on a measured course to gauge progress. It knows the distance and the time it took to travel from A to B, so it easily provides speed (or pace) data. These devices certainly tell you a lot about performance, and they are especially popular with runners. Your speed for a given distance has a lot to do with how well you are performing. It's essentially the same as using a stopwatch on a measured course. There's no doubt that the last-place finisher and the winner of a race had different speeds.

The downside of speed-and-distance devices is that they are currently unable to make adjustments for terrain and course surfaces. Speed as reported in miles per hour (or pace as minutes per mile) decreases when climbing and increases when descending. This makes it difficult to gauge intensity during a workout. In the near future, these devices will "normalize" hill data and report it as the equivalent of speed on a flat course. TrainingPeaks (www.trainingpeaks.com) software can do this during analysis, but that doesn't do you any good while in the middle of a workout. The course surface is also important to speed. Whether you are running, cycling, or Nordic skiing, you will go more slowly on a soft surface such as sand or slushy snow. Unfortunately, neither the speed-and-distance device nor the analysis software can differentiate between surfaces. That's also unlikely in the near future. So, at least for right now, a speed-and-distance device works best on flat, firm courses.

Although power meters have been around since the late 1980s, they've become popular among cyclists only since the early 2000s. The power meter is the ultimate tool for measuring performance. In the not-too-distant future, power meters will take the place of speed-and-distance devices for running and other sports because they are fully capable of reporting performance on hills, into or with the wind, and on soft or firm surfaces. Unfortunately, they are the most expensive of the tools currently available, although prices are beginning to drop.

A power meter measures the force you apply and the rate at which you apply it. On a bike, that means how big your selected gear is and how quickly you turn the cranks. As either increases with the other staying constant, power increases. In nondrafting events such as time trials, power is directly related to time. The only variable is the combined weight of the athlete and the equipment. This is often normalized for comparison by reporting power relative to weight, as in *watts per kilogram*.

While the power meter is currently the ultimate tool for measuring performance, it is available today only for cycling sports and ergometers, such as rowing machines. A few companies have reportedly been working on power meters for other sports, with the most likely being for running, where the device will be built into shoes. When reliable power measurement arrives for running, it will revolutionize the sport as well as any other sport for which it may be adapted.

You likely have one or more of these sport measurement tools and know how to use it. How can you use it to accurately measure fitness changes in training? Let's take a look at three simple tests to gauge your improvement in regard to being fitter and faster.

Aerobic-Threshold Test

In Chapter 4 I introduced the idea of comparing output (speed, pace, or power) with input (effort or heart rate) to find something called the efficiency factor (EF). There it was suggested as a way of determining how your interval workouts are progressing. The same method is especially useful in determining changes in aerobic fitness from week to week by measuring the EF of your aerobic threshold.

If you know your lactate threshold heart rate based on a lab test or a 20-minute test (described later in the section titled "Lactate Threshold Test"), subtract 30 beats per minute (bpm) for a rough estimate of your aerobic threshold. For athletes using my heart rate zone system, that will place your aerobic threshold around upper zone 1 or lower zone 2. Of course, you can get a much more accurate estimate if you get tested in a lab.

Knowing this, all you need to gauge aerobic threshold progress is to measure EF using your heart rate monitor along with either a stopwatch, a speed-and-distance device, or a power meter. Efficiency—how much effort or energy it takes to produce a particular speed or power—is one of the best indicators of fitness for endurance athletes. Let me refresh your memory on how to measure EF; then we'll apply it to your aerobic threshold.

The starting point when measuring training progress is to control as many potential performance-affecting variables as possible. You need to gather lots of data, which means that you need to record EF over the

TABLE 5.1. **Example of Efficiency Factor Determination Using a Stopwatch or Speed-and-Distance Device**

Average heart rate (bpm)	125
Average speed (mph)	7.5 (to convert pace to speed, divide 60 by pace in minutes; e.g., an 8-minute pace is 60 ÷ 8 = 7.5 mph)
Average speed (yards/min)	220 (7.5 × 1,760 yards in a mile ÷ 60, the number of minutes in an hour)
Efficiency factor	1.76 (220 ÷ 125)

Note: The 3-mile test portion (following a warm-up) is done at the aerobic threshold with an average heart rate of 125 bpm.

TABLE 5.2. **Example of Efficiency Factor Determination Using a Power Meter**

Average heart rate (bpm)	125
Normalized power (watts)	150
Efficiency factor	1.2 (150 ÷ 125)

Note: The 30-minute test portion (following a warm-up) is done at the aerobic threshold with an average heart rate of 125 bpm.

course of several workouts done over several weeks. The sessions to be compared should be quite similar in terms of the course, duration, and especially intensity. Your aerobic-threshold heart rate is the perfect intensity for measuring EF during this test. For example, once a week, perform an aerobic-threshold workout on the same course, with the same warm-up and in the same heart rate range (use your aerobic-threshold heart rate plus or minus 2 bpm) for the test portion. The test portion of the workout may take several minutes to a few hours to complete, depending upon the event for which you are training. An Ironman triathlon and a 5K running race, though both are endurance events, have nowhere near the same endurance demands, so the workouts will be of different durations.

When done, divide your average speed (in yards per minute) or Normalized Power (see my book *The Power Meter Handbook* for an explanation of this) for the test portion of the workout by your average heart rate for the same portion. Table 5.1 provides an example of how to calculate EF using a stopwatch or a speed-and-distance device for runners, swimmers, and Nordic skiers. For cyclists or rowers using a power meter, see Table 5.2 for an example.

EF is based on the simple principle that as fitness improves, you go faster (or produce more power) at a given heart rate.[14] Therefore, as your

TABLE 5.3. **Example of the Progression of the Efficiency Factor at Aerobic Threshold for a Road Cyclist Using a Power Meter and Heart Rate Monitor**

WEEK	NORMALIZED POWER (NP)	AVERAGE HEART RATE (AHR)	EFFICIENCY FACTOR (NP/AHR)
1	166	121	1.37
2	170	123	1.38
3	163	123	1.33
4	168	124	1.35
5	172	123	1.40
6	175	125	1.40
7	176	124	1.42
8	177	125	1.41

EF increases, your aerobic fitness likewise increases. The opposite is also true: As EF decreases, aerobic fitness goes with it.

But because you are a human and not a robot, the changes won't always be for the better, even though your fitness is improving. There are simply too many variables that can't be controlled in the daily life of a human. Table 5.3 offers an example of the EF for a cyclist I coached. He rode for 1 hour once a week at a standard aerobic-threshold heart rate range between 121 and 125 bpm, and he also used a power meter. His EF results were derived from several quite similar workouts conducted over an eight-week period.

Note that this rider's EF changes were not always positive. In weeks 3 and 8, his EF decreased slightly. These drops could be the result of changes in sleep, diet, weather, traffic, work-related distress, or a myriad of other factors. Over the course of the eight weeks, though, he did see significant improvement. My point is that testing is not perfect. What you are looking for are trends with similar conditions over time. A generally rising EF is a good sign that your aerobic fitness is improving.

Aerobic-Capacity Test

In Chapter 3 you read that your speed or power at aerobic capacity (VO_2max) can be maintained for about 5 minutes. That means you can self-conduct a field test to measure changes without having to go to a lab and pay for expensive testing using sophisticated equipment. I'd recommend testing your aerobic capacity every three to six weeks throughout the training season.

This test is best done when you are rested and have recovered from the previous several days of training. That means the best time to test is after a few days of R&R. In Chapter 6, I'll show you how to design your training to include R&R breaks from hard training.

I RECOMMEND TESTING your aerobic capacity every three to six weeks throughout the training season.

Here's how to do the test if you are using a speed-and-distance device or a power meter. Following a warm-up, go as fast as you can on a standard course for 5 minutes. The course may be flat, or it can have a continuous upgrade. It is best that it not be a rolling course with both up- and downhill sections. Use the same course every time you test. The first few times athletes do this test, they almost always start too fast. It's best to start slightly slower than you think is possible and speed up in the latter half.

If you don't have a speed-and-distance device or a power meter and are using a stopwatch, you need make only one slight change. Instead of using time as the fixed variable, you'll keep the distance constant. So measure a section of the course that you think will take about 5 minutes, and mark the start and finish points. Again, use the same course every time you test, and don't start out too fast.

Of course, what you should see happen over time is that your speed or power for 5 minutes, or your time on a measured course, improves. This is a good indicator that your fitness, especially your aerobic capacity, is improving. That's one of the key markers of performance in senior athletes, as research has shown it to be the predictor of fitness that declines the fastest with aging.

Lactate-Threshold Test

This lactate-threshold test is quite similar to the 5-minute test except that it's longer. It serves as an indicator of how your lactate-threshold fitness, as described in Chapter 3, is progressing. Lactate threshold is considered the second-most-likely predictor of fitness to decline with aging, so it is important to track accurately and often.

This test is done exactly like the five-minute aerobic-capacity test except that this one involves going fast for 20 minutes, or going fast on a measured course that takes about 20 minutes. As with the shorter test, do this test once every three to six weeks following an R&R break from hard training. It's best that you use the same course every time you do this test. The course should be either flat or slightly uphill; don't use a course that has significant downhill sections. As in the 5-minute test, improved fitness is indicated by a greater average speed or higher power over 20 minutes, or by a faster time on a standard, measured course that takes about 20 minutes to complete.

The 20-minute test may be used to estimate your Functional Threshold Power (FTPo) or Functional Threshold Pace (FTPa). For FTPo, subtract 5 percent from your Normalized Power for the test. For FTPa, convert pace to speed by dividing 60 by your average 1-mile pace for the test. Again, subtract 5 percent to estimate FTPa. In a similar manner, you can get a good approximation of your lactate-threshold heart rate by subtracting 5 percent from your average heart rate for the 20 minutes.

These two tests may both be done within the same workout or on separate days. If doing them on the same day, do the 5-minute test first, with a long recovery following it before starting the 20-minute test. Of course, what you'd like to see is greater speed or power, or a faster time, any of which indicate that your fitness is improving.

The key principle in the testing described above is this: That which is measured improves. By observing and recording your EF in your training journal on a weekly basis and your aerobic capacity and lactate-threshold test results every few weeks, you'll be keenly aware of your training and how it is impacting your fitness. That means you can make training corrections whenever it becomes apparent that things aren't going as planned. You may, for example, find with testing that your EF is coming along quite well, but your aerobic capacity is not improving at all. That may lead you to make changes in your training to include more aerobic-capacity interval workouts. Without accurate feedback, you may not find out until race day.

Basic Training

The purpose of this chapter was to scare you a bit. While I've been proposing all along that you do high-intensity training with aerobic-capacity intervals and heavy-load strength training, I want you to fully realize that such training is risky. The most common risk for the senior athlete is a breakdown due to injury. But overtraining is also possible, and it occurs now with a much lower training load than when you were a youngster.

Greed regarding the reward of a given workout or period of training is what most often leads to such breakdowns and lost training. For the senior athlete, not training means that the rate at which aerobic capacity and muscle mass are lost accelerates. What may have been a half percentage point lost per year now doubles (or worse). For the oldest senior athletes, if the lost training time from such a breakdown is significant, it may not be possible to regain the losses once training is resumed. The key to preventing such losses is moderation—conservative starting levels for intervals and weight lifting and cautious progression going forward. Do somewhat less than you think is possible at the time. If in doubt, leave it out. Don't do the last interval if you feel as if you have only one left in you. Stop short of the last rep in the weight room, regardless of what the plan may call for.

It's also possible to train too moderately to avoid risk and therefore end up not reaping the reward. That's where testing comes in. By frequently and regularly measuring your EF, aerobic capacity, and lactate threshold, you will know whether or not your fitness is progressing. If these markers show improvement, then your fitness is on course for a good race performance. If they aren't, then you can make appropriate adjustments in your training.

In the next chapter I'll bring many of the loose ends together to show you how to create a training plan that matches your unique needs.

ADVANCED TRAINING

It's not what you once did that counts the most, but what you keep doing.
—JOHNNY KELLEY

The starting point for high performance, once you have a goal, is creating a long-term training plan. That may sound tedious and boring. This one small step, however, is perhaps the most important thing you can do to return your fitness to where it was when you were a much younger athlete. By establishing a plan for your season, especially a standard weekly routine, you'll take a huge step toward increasing aerobic capacity and muscle mass. You've been reading about these two aging limiters for several chapters. Now it's finally time to do something about them.

Seasonal planning includes what was covered in Chapters 4 and 5. Those chapters introduced you to a general concept of how to train using high-intensity workouts—intervals and weight lifting. Now it's time for you to make decisions about when, including how frequently, to do such workouts and to determine the workloads for each. This takes us to the next step in once again becoming fast: creating a plan.

The process of planning goes well beyond moderation, consistency, risk, and reward. These are critical, but now it's time to blend "need to" with "how to." With your newfound *philosophy* of moderation in place, the next step is to develop a *methodology* for training. This chapter takes you from pie-in-the-sky academic thinking to real-life training. What that means is something I'm sure you've heard of previously, since you're a serious athlete: periodization.

WITH YOUR newfound **philosophy** of moderation in place, the next step is to develop a **methodology** for training.

Successful periodization is based entirely on the individual athlete—you. There isn't just one way to train that works for all senior athletes in all situations. We don't all have the same needs. For example, the newer someone is to sport, the more likely he or she is to improve performance by simply training frequently. Planning is simple: Get out the door and do it a few times each week. After a year or so, the next common step for beginners in their training progression is to increase the durations of their workouts. That's just slightly more complex. This introduces a new level of stress and produces nice gains in fitness—for a while.

For the highly experienced veteran athlete, however, solely doing frequent and long training sessions offers little in the way of reward. High-intensity training along with frequent and long-duration sessions is much more beneficial, albeit also more risky. Mixing all of these makes for an intricate training plan. In doing so, there are a couple of other things to consider beyond moderation and risk.

While experience plays an important role in determining the interplay of training frequency, duration, and intensity, there is certainly more to training. Your unique situation must always be considered when designing a training program. In addition to your experience, you should also take into account the intricacies of your sport, prior training methods, health, sensitivity to training stress, risk of injury, time available for training, the goal event you are preparing for, and the abilities and experience of your training partners. In addition to these, you must consider the environmental factors of where you live and train, such as altitude, terrain, weather, equipment, or venue availability. Even if aerobic-capacity and strength training to increase muscle mass are physiologically the right areas of training for you, some of these environmental factors may interfere with your progression when designing and following a training plan.

By now you should thoroughly understand the benefits of high-intensity intervals and strength training for you as a senior athlete. And as I emphasized in the previous chapter, it's imperative that you take into consideration the risks associated with such training. So if you are to train as I've proposed, you must somehow decrease the risk. The way to do this is to be cautious with your training load starting points, careful with the rate at which you increase them, and conservative with how frequently you perform such workouts. That means having a plan and being flexible in carrying it out.

Dose and Density

Fitness results from training, and training is quite simple. There are only two components.

$$\text{Training} = \text{Stress} + \text{Recovery}$$

Getting the mix of these two right is not so simple, however. In this chapter we will further examine the stress part of the equation, and in Chapter 7 we'll delve into recovery.

It's not easy to determine how great your training stress should be in order to produce fitness, especially while making changes such as including more high intensity in your workouts. There are two common mistakes made by serious athletes, regardless of age, when they enthusiastically make the shift toward more intensity-based stress. They make the workouts too hard, and they space them too closely together. This combination is certain to produce a breakdown such as an injury, illness, or even overtraining.

The solution to this training dilemma brings us to the twin topics of "dose" and "density." Dose has to do with how great the training load is on any given day. High intensity is high dose. High duration is likewise high dose. On the other side of the coin, low intensity and duration are low dose.

Density is how many high-dose workouts you do in a given period of time, such as a week. The older you are, the less dense your training should probably be. A 30-year-old athlete can typically manage more density than a 60-year-old can. As age increases, the density of training typically needs to decrease. The same is true for dose.

Dose is the controlling variable, and density is adjusted in response to it. As dose rises, meaning the individual workouts become harder, density must decrease to allow for recovery and to avoid breakdown. Conversely, as dose decreases, density can increase. Later in this chapter, when we get into periodization, you will see this interplay at work. And as you begin to train as suggested later in this chapter, it will make perfect sense to you.

While both dose and density are concerns of the senior athlete, I've found that density becomes the one that gives us the most trouble as we get older. That is due to our slower rate of recovery following high-dose workouts. We can generally do a high-dose session, perhaps even as hard as when we were much younger, but we can't do several of them in a few days' time. We need more recovery than younger athletes do after similar workouts.

Like the pause between the notes in a song, inserting recovery days between high-dose workouts gives training a rhythm (and we'll discuss recovery in Chapter 7). Inserting breaks ensures that the density is manageable. As with all things related to recovery—and just about everything else when talking about aging—we each have unique requirements, so I can't tell you exactly what your dose and density should be. You'll have to figure that out for yourself based on experience and perhaps even trial and error. But I can help you get started down the right path.

Let's begin by reviewing the workout dosage for the high-intensity workouts you've been reading about. In the following "Optimal Density Training" section, you'll consider suggestions for the frequency of your high-dose workouts.

Table 6.1 provides examples of high-, moderate-, and low-dose versions of aerobic-capacity, lactate-threshold, aerobic-threshold, and strength workouts.

High-Dose Workouts

Workouts are the source of training stress. For the senior athlete, these are aerobic-capacity intervals or fartlek, lactate-threshold intervals, aerobic-threshold steady-states, and heavy-load weight lifting. A uniquely individualized blend of these will produce the potential for a high level of fitness over the course of a few weeks. For experienced athletes, the key to successful fitness development in these is the intensity of each. Get the intensity right and faster racing is almost guaranteed.

Of nearly equal importance is how long the recoveries should last after each of the intervals and reps. You've read about each of these key workouts in previous chapters, but to ensure that you fully understand each before plugging them into a plan, let's do a quick review.

The Aerobic-Capacity Interval Workout

You'll recall that the purpose of this workout is to increase your aerobic capacity ($\dot{V}O_2$max)—your body's ability to use oxygen to produce energy. The higher your aerobic capacity, the greater your potential for speed. To revive your aerobic capacity, which may be in hibernation after several years of inattention, you must do workouts at or near your aerobic-capacity intensity. That's the highest intensity you can maintain for about 5 minutes in an all-out effort. In fact, as explained in earlier chapters, that's the best way to determine this workout's intensity short of paying to have an aerobic-capacity test done in a lab. Simply do a 5-minute time trial (see Chapter 5 for the details). Your average pace, speed, or power for this test is the intensity to be used in aerobic-capacity workouts.

Note that these workouts must be done "at or near" your aerobic-capacity intensity. The intensity can range from right at aerobic capacity to about 10 percent less, so you've got some wiggle room. There is no reason, however, to exceed this intensity range. All you'll accomplish by doing so is to increase your risk of breakdown while prolonging recovery in the following hours and days.

Table 6.1 suggests that you do intervals for this workout that range from 30 seconds to 3 minutes. This is a fairly typical range that has been shown to be quite effective for boosting this specific type of fitness.[1] The interval durations listed there are only suggestions; they can be changed. A high-dose session could just as well be 30 × 30 seconds as the suggested 5 × 3 minutes. Both make for a workout with 15 minutes of total interval time—the *most* I'd recommend you do. The longer intervals may have a slight advantage in terms of fitness gains, but doing what you find works best for you, both physically and mentally, is the key to success.

So how do you gauge the intensity of aerobic capacity when doing these intervals? Getting the intensity much too high or way too low will sabotage

TABLE 6.1. **Suggested Training Details for High-, Moderate-, and Low-Dose Workouts**

WORKOUT TYPE	HIGH DOSE	MODERATE DOSE	LOW DOSE
Aerobic-capacity intervals Intensity at or slightly below VO$_2$max speed/power/perceived exertion	5 × 2.5 min (2.5 min recoveries) 5 × 3 min (3 min recoveries)	6 × 1.5 min (1.5 min recoveries) 5 × 2 min (2 min recoveries)	10 × 30 sec (30 sec recoveries) 7 × 1 min (1 min recoveries)
Lactate-threshold intervals Intensity: 90–95% of LTHR* or 88–93% of FTP** speed/power.	3 × 12 min (3 min 15 sec recoveries) 2 × 20 min (5 min recoveries)	3 × 8 min (2.5 min recoveries) 3 × 10 min (3 min recoveries)	3 × 5 min (90 sec recoveries) 3 × 6 min (2 min recoveries)
Aerobic threshold Intensity: continuous and steady at about 30 bpm < LTHR* ± 2 bpm. Duration: dependent on goal event.	2–4 hr	1–2 hr	30 min–1 hr
Weight lifting Simulate the movements of your sport with full recoveries after each set. Low reps mean high loads.	7–9 reps 3–6 reps	13–15 reps 10–12 reps	20–30 reps 16–19 reps

* Lactate-threshold heart rate; ** Functional Threshold Power
Note: Each workout is preceded by a warm-up and followed by a cooldown.

the workout. There are several ways to gauge intensity: speed or pace, heart rate, power, and perceived exertion. Of these, the least effective is heart rate. When doing intervals as short as 30 seconds to 3 minutes, heart rate lags well behind the effort being produced and may not achieve the aerobic capacity (or VO$_2$max) zone until very late in the interval, if at all.

What the athlete typically does when using a heart rate monitor with these intervals is to start much too fast in an attempt to get heart rate to rise quickly and then, once heart rate is up, slow down to stabilize it. This is just the opposite of what should be done in an interval workout.

Short of doing the interval at a steady speed, the best way of pacing each is to start slightly easier than aerobic capacity—by around 10 percent—and then increase the intensity as the interval progresses. You'll be better off using perceived exertion than heart rate for this workout. On a scale of 1 (low) to 10 (high), your perceived exertion for this workout should be an 8 or 9. That is pretty challenging. Power and pace (or speed) are by far the most effective ways to gauge interval intensity.

LIKE THE PAUSE between the notes in a song, inserting recovery days between high-dose workouts gives training a rhythm.

As a quick summary, the intervals suggested here are 30 seconds to 3 minutes long with equal recovery durations after each (you can find aerobic-capacity workout details in Appendix A). The reason for the equal recoveries is to give your body a chance to recover before doing the next one.[2] If you are new to aerobic-capacity intervals, you may even make the recoveries somewhat longer than the previous work interval to ensure that you have recovered before starting the next one.

During each of these slow and easy recoveries, you must determine how you are handling the stress. It's far better to stop short of the scheduled number of intervals if something doesn't feel right than to press on and end up extremely sore for several days, or even injured.

For the aerobic-capacity workout, aim for a total of 5 to 15 minutes of combined interval time within a session, depending on the dose size you've decided to use. If it's been a while since you last did such high-intensity intervals, start with a low dose such as 10 × 30 seconds. If it's been years since you trained this way, it may even be wise to do less than 5 minutes of total interval time in one session. Always remember moderation. Be especially cautious at first.

As the season progresses and supercompensation works its magic, you will be able to increase the dosage by doing longer intervals with more total interval time within a session. But don't force the progression to happen quickly. Pay attention to how you feel during and after each of these workouts, and progress at a moderate rate. A 10 percent increase in combined interval time in each subsequent workout is about right for most senior athletes. If there is any doubt about how well you coped with the previous workout's stress, then keep it the same or even less in the next session and reevaluate after that.

Again, instead of intervals, this workout can be done as fartlek. That means the session is unstructured and based entirely on "feel" for how long the durations are, how intensely you exercise, and when you decide to stop. Such a workout is probably best done after a session or two of structured intervals so that you can refine your sense of how great the stress should be. Aerobic-capacity intervals may be done as hill repeats or even as a group workout that includes several fast portions. The gold standard for this type of training, however, is the structured interval session, as described in Table 6.1 and Appendix A.

As I've mentioned before, high-intensity intervals increase your risk of breakdown, especially from an injury. That's why I suggest you start with a low-dose workout and progress cautiously to higher dosages. An injury will delay your training and set you back in terms of the gains made in slowing the constraints of aging.

I'm often asked, especially by runners, if this workout can be done in an alternate sport due to the risk of injury. This is called "crosstraining," and it can be beneficial, but probably not as much as if you do the workout in your primary sport. Crosstraining, however, may be a great option for the runner who is frequently injured. For example, a runner may want to do this workout on a bike, as these two sports have been shown to be mutually compatible in terms of aerobic-capacity development.[3]

Triathletes may also take advantage of this crosstraining relationship to avoid injury and to make training density more manageable. It's the old "two birds with one stone" concept. Doing aerobic-capacity intervals on a bike will produce better running aerobic capacity, and vice versa.

How about the crosstraining effect for swimming? Unfortunately, intervals done by running or cycling have been shown to be of *no* benefit to swimming.[4] If you're a triathlete, doing bike or run intervals won't measurably boost your swim aerobic capacity. And if your sport is swimming, do the intervals in the pool, not on a bike or a run.

The Lactate-Threshold Interval Workout

Research tells us that aerobic-capacity intervals improve not only your VO_2max but also your lactate threshold[5] and probably even your economy.[6] Those are all three of the markers of fitness you read about in Chapter 3. That's a lot of bang for your buck. But if aerobic capacity is not a fitness limiter for you, it's likely that lactate threshold is restricting your performance gains.

About the only way you would know with any degree of certainty that lactate threshold is restricting your performance would be if you had your aerobic capacity tested in a lab regularly for several years and found that your VO_2max remained consistently high, with an average annual decline of less than 0.5 percent. In that case, doing lots of aerobic-capacity interval training is probably unnecessary. Something else is obviously working out well for your aerobic capacity. Including additional training stress is

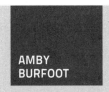

**AMBY
BURFOOT**

Recovery and Crosstraining

In April 2014 I finished the Boston Marathon 49 years after my first Boston run in 1965. The previous Thanksgiving, I completed an annual "Turkey Trot" 5-miler in Manchester, Connecticut, for the 51st year in a row.

You don't manage these kinds of longevity feats unless you have a healthy relationship with injuries. I do, and I believe I have actually gotten wiser as I've grown older. That said, I've also been lucky. None of us are immune to injuries, and if you get one at the wrong time . . . well, that's a race you're not going to do.

At least, not if you're smart. Running a race while injured tops my list of stupid runner tricks. I suppose if I had ever made it to the Olympics, which I didn't, I would have been tempted to race no matter what. Short of the Olympics, I can't think of another event that anyone should run while injured. It's just not worth the risk of making the injury more severe and longer-lasting.

What's at the top of my intelligent injury-prevention tricks? That's easy. Take days off at regular intervals, and particularly when you first notice a nagging pain. This one took me a while to learn. When I was young and fast, I thought I was bulletproof. I believed I could run and run and not get injured. I learned otherwise when I developed a metatarsal fracture.

Next, I believed that I could "run through" modest pain. I was obsessed with maintaining a high weekly training mileage; I was willing to slow down but not to skip runs. To be honest, this worked on occasion. But other times it didn't, and I lost more training time to the resulting injuries than what I "saved" by running through mild discomfort.

As I aged into a masters competitor, I mostly made my peace with injuries. I realized I didn't need to be in top shape every single day— »

Continued

in fact, couldn't be—so I accepted the wisdom of several days off whenever I felt an unusual and unwelcome twinge. Nowadays, I take three days off from running when I sense an impending injury.

Most of the time, I can use my recumbent bike at home without pain. This of course is the other great trick that masters athletes must accept: more crosstraining. I do about 65 percent of my weekly exercise on the recumbent bike. It's hardly even training. I just pedal easily for 40 to 60 minutes while reading a book or magazine.

I've never been one to stretch and only recently have begun consistent, very simple strength training. I'm dubious that stretching prevents injuries, but I never try to dissuade someone who thinks it does and enjoys the stretching process (which I don't). It makes sense to me that appropriate strength and balance training could prevent some injuries.

At age 68, and about 105,000 total lifetime miles, my only goal is to keep on keeping on. I'd do just about anything to prevent a running injury . . . except stop running entirely. I hope that my good luck continues.

risky and more than is apparently needed to boost your lactate threshold. In this situation, you are better off focusing on lactate-threshold intervals and doing only minimal maintenance training for aerobic capacity, meaning low dose and low density.

Another way to determine your own best blend of aerobic-capacity and lactate-threshold training is to consider the type of events for which you are training. Events that take less than 30 minutes or so to complete are likely to benefit more from aerobic-capacity training than from lactate-threshold intervals. So the mix of the two might best be shifted in favor of shorter, more intense intervals. If your most important races are typically 30 minutes to about 2 hours long, then your training focus is better placed on lactate threshold, as aerobic capacity is somewhat less critical to your success as race duration increases. Bicycle road racing may be the exception to this general rule, since even in the longest races the outcomes are determined by brief episodes of very high intensity. For cycling, focusing on aerobic capacity is likely to be important regardless of race duration.

What about training for events that take longer than 2 hours? The proper blend of aerobic-capacity and lactate-threshold intervals would still favor the latter, but the most critical type of training would shift in favor of the aerobic-threshold workout. The longer the event duration, the greater this shift should be. While this type of training was introduced in Chapter 5, we haven't examined it very closely because it isn't tied to any of the physiological declines we experience with aging. But when it comes to endurance training for long events, it is still something all senior athletes should include in their training. The only question is, how much of such training should be done? Hold on to that thought, as we'll return to the topic soon.

First, let's return to lactate-threshold intervals.

As you can see in Table 6.1, lactate-threshold intervals are done at a lower intensity and are considerably longer than intervals done for aerobic-capacity development. As with aerobic-capacity intervals, the best intensity for lactate-threshold intervals is *at or slightly below* your lactate-threshold intensity.

To determine your lactate-threshold intensity, you can do a lab test, or, less expensively, you can do a 20-minute time trial, as described in Appendix B. As with the 5-minute aerobic-capacity test, your lactate threshold is specific to each discipline. So if you are a triathlete, you need to complete a test in each sport.

By subtracting 5 percent from your average speed or power found in that test, you know how to gauge lactate-threshold intensity for your intervals. Since the intervals are long, this type of interval training can be done effectively using a heart rate monitor. Your average heart rate minus 5 percent for the entire 20-minute time trial is a pretty good predictor of lactate-threshold heart rate. So you could do the lactate-threshold intervals at that calculated heart rate or as much as *another* 5 percent lower.

If you prefer to do intervals based on perceived exertion rather than by using an intensity-measuring device such as a heart rate monitor, GPS, accelerometer, or power meter, then the effort should feel like a 6 or 7 on a scale of 1 (low) to 10 (high).

Besides intensity, the other key elements of the lactate-threshold workout are the durations of the intervals and the durations of the slow and easy recoveries. Long intervals, as suggested in Table 6.1, are best for developing such fitness.[7] The purpose of the long interval is to cause a slight rise in blood lactate, indicating that hydrogen ions are accumulating and increasing the acidity of the working muscles, which gradually reduces their power. The recoveries are short to ensure that the hydrogen ions are not completely removed by the time you start the next interval. To be short, the recovery duration should be about one-fourth as long as the preceding interval.

Over the course of a few such long intervals with short recoveries, the acidity gradually accumulates, placing slowly increasing stress on the working muscles. During your eventual rest, your body will respond (remember supercompensation from Chapter 5?) by going through changes that result in adaption to the stress. You will become better at tolerating the acid and, more importantly, more effective at buffering it. If the recoveries between the intervals are overly long, the acid will be mostly flushed from the muscles by the time of the next interval, and that will diminish your body's need to adapt. That in turn will result in little or no change in performance. That's why I recommend long intervals done at or near lactate threshold with short recoveries.

Can you effectively crosstrain with lactate-threshold intervals by doing them in a sport other than your primary one? Research is lacking in this area, so we don't have data to back up such an approach. My sense is that crosstraining here is not as effective as it was for aerobic capacity because as the intensity of training decreases, the focus of fitness shifts more toward the muscles and away from the central systems such as the heart's stroke volume. Muscle recruitment is highly specific to the sport. Therefore, I believe your lactate-threshold training should be done only in your primary sport. For example, runners should do running workouts to fully reap the benefits of lactate-threshold training because the risk of a running injury is much lower than in aerobic-capacity training. Likewise, triathletes should do lactate-threshold intervals in each of their three sports.

The Aerobic-Threshold Workout

In Chapter 5 I introduced a new type of workout, one that may be similar to what you already do a lot of—long, slow distance (LSD). The main difference is that what I suggest is not really "slow" in the way that LSD is normally done. In fact, one of the outcomes of this type of workout is that your speed becomes increasingly faster at a low effort. It could be called "long, moderate distance" or "long, *steady* distance." But instead we call it the "aerobic-threshold" workout.

Aerobic-threshold training isn't directly linked to reversing or slowing the ravages of aging, as aerobic-capacity intervals are. This workout is exclusively about endurance performance. And since that's what this chapter is about, we need to review it.

With the other two types of critical workouts I've explained so far—aerobic-capacity and lactate-threshold intervals—you train at or near either your aerobic capacity or your lactate threshold. Now we're going to apply the same principle to improving your aerobic threshold. (A word of caution: Don't confuse "aerobic threshold" with "anaerobic threshold," which is another common term for what we've been calling the "lactate threshold." The *aerobic* threshold occurs at a much lower intensity.) This is an important intensity that, as we'll see shortly, has a lot to do with how efficiently you use your body's fuel while exercising.

Let's start by reviewing the basics of fuel utilization during endurance exercise.

One of the primary purposes of endurance training is to boost your body's ability to use stored body fat for fuel instead of glycogen. Your body's supply of glycogen, its storage form of carbohydrate, is extremely limited compared with its supply of fat. Even the skinniest endurance athlete has enough energy stored in the body as blubber to exercise continuously for days. But that same athlete has only enough glycogen to exercise vigorously for about 2 hours. So one of the purposes of training is to increase your body's reliance on stored fat while sparing glycogen. All endurance workouts, including aerobic-capacity and lactate-threshold intervals, help this to happen. But aerobic-threshold workouts are the most effective for inducing this critical change.

Besides becoming better at using fat for fuel, you gain several other benefits from training at or near your aerobic threshold. This type of training relies almost exclusively on your slow-twitch muscle fibers—your endurance muscles—so most of the beneficial changes take place there. When you train frequently at your aerobic threshold, your slow-twitch muscles adapt by developing more capillaries. This in turn creates more delivery pathways for blood, and therefore oxygen and fuel.[8] The fuel, in this case, is fat.

Although the primary muscles used for this workout are slow twitch, a few fast-twitch, or power muscles, are also recruited to help out when fatigue eventually appears. The fast-twitch muscles recruited are the ones that are most similar to the slow twitchers. They already have some endurance characteristics. When these primarily power-related muscles are called into action to assist as fatigue sets in during the aerobic-threshold workout, they become better at using oxygen to produce energy from fat. So these fast-twitch muscles eventually supercompensate by taking on even more of the characteristics of your primary endurance muscles.[9] That's a good thing, as it improves your endurance.

In addition, as a result of the aerobic-threshold workout, all of the recruited muscles develop more aerobic enzymes, the chemicals that help produce energy from oxygen and fat.[10] As an added bonus of these workouts, the kidneys begin to create more of the hormone erythropoietin (EPO), which stimulates red-blood-cell production. More red blood cells mean more oxygen-carrying capacity to the muscles.[11]

Taken together, these benefits are huge for your endurance performance. And they all result from one type of activity—the long, moderate-intensity, steady, aerobic-threshold workout. As you'll see later on, this will become one of the staples of your training, not to slow aging but to improve performance while also improving your ability to burn body fat.

These adaptations are all tremendously important physiological changes. Nevertheless, the one we remain most focused on is the use of body blubber for fuel in order to spare your limited glycogen stores. Your capability to primarily burn fat is dependent on several other factors, such as gender (women are more inclined to use fat than men), fitness (the greater the fitness, the more fat is used), and chronic diet.[12] We'll return with much greater detail to this last factor in Chapter 8.

Essentially, when you do a lot of aerobic-threshold training, you are teaching your body to use fat for fuel. When you perform aerobic-capacity or lactate-threshold interval sessions, most of the fuel comes from your limited reserves of glycogen, especially if your diet is high in carbohydrate (more on this topic in Chapter 8). At below 60 percent of aerobic capacity, the intensity for aerobic-threshold development, fat becomes the dominant fuel.[13] So that is the intensity you need to use for this workout. Many athletes feel that this is too easy, and so they increase the intensity to something approaching or even exceeding 70 percent. That defeats the workout's purpose and is not as effective at improving your fat burning.

This all sounds great, but how exactly do you do an aerobic-threshold workout? The two keys are, as always, intensity and duration. This is a workout that can be done very nicely using a heart rate monitor to gauge intensity. We just need to identify the proper heart rate. Chapter 5 described this, but it's important enough that we will review it again now.

At 60 percent of your aerobic capacity, as mentioned earlier, you are exercising at roughly 70 percent of your maximum heart rate. But don't worry about finding that number. For most experienced and dedicated athletes, the aerobic threshold is about 30 beats per minute below your lactate-threshold heart rate. That's the intensity you discovered when preparing to do lactate-threshold intervals. You may have found it by having a lab test done or by simply doing a 20-minute time trial and then subtracting 5 percent from the time trial's average heart rate. Now subtract an additional 30 bpm, and you have a good estimate of your aerobic threshold. (If you are using my heart rate zone system, the aerobic threshold occurs roughly at the zone 2 threshold—slightly above or slightly below.)

Next, add and subtract 2 bpm, and you have a 5-beat aerobic-threshold zone. For example, if your lactate-threshold heart rate was found to be 150, subtracting 30 predicts an aerobic-threshold heart rate of 120. Adding and subtracting 2 produces a training range of 118 to 122. This range will remain consistent throughout the season even as your fitness improves.

There is a lot of estimating going on here, which always opens the door for error. A much more precise way to determine your aerobic-threshold intensity is to undertake a VO_2max test conducted in a lab, health club, or sporting-goods store or by a coach in your sport. While it's a bit expensive, the test will establish not only your aerobic threshold but also your aerobic capacity and lactate (or anaerobic) threshold. Make sure the technician knows what data you want before you start the test.

Since aerobic-threshold intensity is much lower than that of the other workouts you've read about here, the dosage for the aerobic-threshold workout results primarily from its duration. In Table 6.1 you can see that, compared with the other workouts, this one is quite long. It is truly an *endurance* workout.

So how do you determine the aerobic-threshold workout duration that is appropriate for you? It comes down to the expected duration of the event for which you are training. With that in mind, examine Table 6.2 to see how long your aerobic-threshold workouts should be. Start in the top row by finding how long you expect your event to take. Beneath that you will find the suggested time range for your aerobic-threshold workouts. For example, if your race is expected to take about 3 hours, it is in the "2–4 hr" range. Below that you can see that the aerobic-threshold workout duration is "1–2 hr."

Continuing with the example of a projected 3-hour event time, the length of your aerobic-threshold workouts would be 1 to 2 hours. But that

TABLE 6.2. **Duration of Aerobic-Threshold Workout Based on Goal Event's Duration**

Duration of goal event	>4 hr	2–4 hr	<2 hr
Aerobic-threshold workout duration	2–4 hr	1–2 hr	30 min–1 hr

doesn't mean that the first time you do this workout, you should start in this range. Since this workout is done almost year-round, you should have lots of time to build aerobic endurance, which is good because it comes slowly. I suggest starting with a 30-minute workout and gradually increasing it every few weeks until you achieve the upper end of the goal duration—2 hours. Then continue to repeat this longest duration frequently in the last few weeks before your event. Later in this chapter we'll come back to what "frequently" and "the last few weeks" mean.

The aerobic-threshold session not only improves endurance performance but also serves as a test for how your aerobic fitness is progressing, as explained in Chapter 5. There you read about the efficiency factor (EF). You'll recall that this involves comparing power or speed (in yards per minute) with heart rate (see Table 5.1 or 5.2). This requires a heart rate monitor and something that measures performance output—a speed-and-distance device (running, swimming, Nordic skiing) or a power meter (cycling, indoor rowing). If you don't have these devices, you are left to guess how well you are progressing.

The Strength Workout

There are two reasons you should do high-load strength training workouts year round. The first is that it has been shown in most of the research to improve performance in experienced athletes, both male and female, in a variety of endurance sports.[14] The second reason is that it has the potential to slow or stop the aging-related loss of muscle mass. That's largely because lifting weights increases the body's production of muscle-building hormones such as growth hormone, testosterone, and insulin-like growth factor.[15]

In the hours following a strength session, your body is already busily rebuilding the muscles you exercised to make them stronger.[16] You can enhance this rebuilding process by including some protein in a postexercise meal in the form of either a supplement or, preferably, real food.[17] How soon afterward remains open for debate, but I suggest eating at least a protein-enhanced snack within an hour of finishing. How much protein should you take in? Somewhat limited research has shown that about 15 to 20 grams of protein, which is 60 to 80 calories, is adequate for this benefit.[18] If you use a supplement, check the label to see how much is necessary to get this amount. (The topic of protein following exercise is discussed in greater detail in Chapter 8.)

You may be enticed to eat a protein bar after a strength session to meet this need because bars are so convenient, but be aware that the sugar content (a topic we will also dig into much more deeply in Chapter 8) is quite high for most of these. Most protein bars aren't much different than a Snickers candy bar. You're better off eating a meal that includes a good source of protein or, failing that, using a powdered protein supplement.

In my Training Bible book series for road cyclists, triathletes, and mountain bikers, I devote an entire chapter in each to the topic of strength development. The chapters include illustrations of strength exercises that are appropriate for those sports. Given the wide range of endurance sports supported by this book, it's not possible to provide such exercise specifics here. If you are not a cyclist, triathlete, or mountain biker, I advise finding a good resource on this topic for your sport. It could be a book, a trusted blog, a personal trainer who knows your sport, or a coach in your sport. The key is to do exercises that closely mimic your sport's movements. I can, however, suggest a training program, minus the exercises, for you based on the principles I have used with the senior athletes I've coached. Let's start by looking at the four phases I have the athlete go through each season.

TABLE 6.3. **Definition of Strength Training Phases for Senior Endurance Athletes**

PHASES IN ORDER OF SEASONAL PLANNING	PURPOSE OF PHASE	SETS PER WORKOUT	DOSE*
Anatomical Adaptation (AA)	Master the movements of each strength exercise and begin muscular adaptation	2–3	Low
Max Transition (MT)	Transition from low to high loads	3	Moderate
Max Strength (MS)	Develop maximum, sport-specific muscle strength	3	High
Strength Maintenance (SM)	Maintain the strength levels developed in MS	2	1 set moderate + 1 set high

* See Table 6.1.

Taken together, the strength-building phases make up a portion of your periodization plan—the order in which the sets, reps, and loads change to gradually and safely produce greater strength. These must match up with your overall, sport-specific periodization plan. If they are out of sync, the density of your training will probably be too great, which will leave you overly tired most of the time.

Table 6.3 lists the sets and rep-load dose for each of the four strength-training phases. Table 6.4 shows how to include the strength phases in a training plan so that they match up with your overall seasonal periodization. Taken together, these tables lay out your strength-training plan for the season.

I realize that we're getting a bit ahead of ourselves by introducing these tables now, as we won't examine periodization and planning until the following sections of this chapter. I suspect, however, that, like nearly all of the

TABLE 6.4. **Strength Training Progression During the Training Season for Senior Endurance Athletes**

ANNUAL TRAINING PERIOD	PERIOD DURATION	STRENGTH PHASE	SESSIONS PER WEEK
Preparation	1–6 weeks	AA, MT	2
Early Base	3–6 weeks	MS	2
Late Base	3–6 weeks	SM	1
Build	9–12 weeks	SM	1
Peak	1–2 weeks	SM	1
Race	1 week	None	None
Transition	1–4 weeks	AA	1–2

Note: AA = Anatomical Adaptation; MS = Max Strength; MT = Max Transition; SM = Strength Maintenance

older athletes I coach, you are familiar with the topic of periodization planning and would prefer to see the tables in conjunction with the associated text. If you are not familiar with periodization and you find this confusing, come back to this section after you have read the rest of this chapter.

Let's consider how to properly do a strength-building workout. Once or twice a week, depending on the phase, is enough to build and maintain an adequate level of strength while slowing muscle loss.[19] After warming up with an aerobic exercise, such as riding a stationary bike or running slowly on a treadmill, begin the session with the most important and most demanding strength exercise for your sport.[20] The first set should be the lightest load to allow for further warm-up. Increase the load in subsequent sets. Complete the number of sets and reps suggested for the phase you are currently in according to Table 6.4.

The focus of your seasonal strength training should be on the Max Strength (MS) phase. In fact, all the lifting you do in the first two phases is to prepare you for MS, and the phases that follow MS are intended to maintain the strength gains made during MS. This phase is best done in the early Base period of your season, when sport-specific training is of lesser importance. Doing it in the late Base or Build period will have a negative effect on your sport-specific workouts. You'll be too tired and sore to do high-quality training in your sport. I can't emphasize this enough. I often hear from athletes who do the MS phase in the later seasonal periods and are simply incapable of doing workouts in their primary sport with the necessary quality.

After MS, as the focus of training shifts to sport-specific workouts, you will move into the Strength Maintenance (SM) period of training. This is a much less stressful phase with less-frequent workouts and diminished total loading. The sets are now reduced to two per exercise, with one moderate-dose set done as a warm-up, followed by a high-dose set with a heavy load. This one set will maintain your strength at an adequate level[21] without the workload stress being too great to hinder training performance the next day in your endurance workout.

In all of the phases, after each set, rest for 3 to 5 minutes.[22]

I also recommend including core strength training into your strength program to stabilize the torso, hips, and shoulders when making the high-intensity movements of your sport.[23] Again, you may need to seek help from other sources to determine which exercises are best for your sport and how they should be done.

There will undoubtedly be times when you miss a strength session, perhaps even several, due to work, family, or other training interruptions. That's to be expected. You should be able to continue without concern for lost strength so long as you haven't missed more than about two weeks of strength workouts.[24]

Optimal-Density Training

We've now been through nearly all of the workouts that, taken together, make up your training—aerobic-capacity intervals, lactate-threshold intervals, aerobic-endurance steady states, and strength training. The only one we haven't covered is the recovery session. We'll do that in Chapter 7. But with what you now know, it's time to put together an annual training plan. This involves the periodization mentioned above. This is where the density—how frequently you do high-dose workouts—becomes the focus.

There are two concerns in planning for density. If the density of your workouts is too great, meaning the hard sessions are spaced too closely together, then you are likely to break down in some way; you may suffer an injury, illness, burnout, or overtraining. If the density is too low, with unnecessary recovery days, your fitness and race performance will suffer because you'll be undertrained. Given the choice, I'd prefer to see you slightly undertrained than chronically overtrained.

Getting density right is specific to your unique situation. The factors involved include not only the dose of your workouts but also your general lifestyle. If you have a job that is physically or emotionally demanding, density may need adjusting so that the highest-dose workouts have adequate separation between them with plenty of time for recovery. If you go through times when emotional stress is high for any reason, such as a divorce, financial issues, changing jobs, moving, or anything else that upsets you, then the density of training must also be adjusted so that you get more recovery.

Even if you don't have anything in your life that requires making such adjustments, getting the density of training right is always difficult and somewhat of a moving target. Things change in your life from time to time. Trial and error is about the only way to find out what your baseline density should be. Some weeks it will be spot-on, and at other times it will be all wrong. So once you decide on a density plan that fits your current needs, you may still have to tweak it occasionally as the stress in your life ebbs and flows. Later in this chapter I'll suggest some routines to help you plan your season with all of this in mind.

Training Periods

Let's get the planning started by examining the duration, purpose, and details of each training period. Table 6.5 is a summary. Note that the period durations listed are ranges, such as "3–6 weeks" for the early Base period. It's presented as a range because you will undoubtedly have more than one A-priority race in a season. For each subsequent A race, you will repeat many of the periods as you prepare using the somewhat shorter durations.

I recommend preparing and subsequently tapering for no more than three A-priority races in a year. The reason is that tapering in order to be rested for the next A race and then rejuvenating with an extended break from training after the race means giving up some fitness. With more than three A-priority races in an annual season, the amount of tapering and resting becomes too costly. Your fitness would be low too often, and you would likely have too little time to regain fitness before the next race. Doing only two or three A races increases the odds that you will have time to reestablish high fitness levels just in time for the next one.

Why the "period duration" ranges for each period? For the first A race of the year, it's usually best to do the longer suggested period durations to reap the full fitness benefits. But for each subsequent A race, you won't need as much time because your fitness will be greater; in these cases, the shorter durations are appropriate. In other words, race readiness comes back more quickly even with less time devoted to it as the season progresses. Also, it's unlikely that for these subsequent A races you need to return to any period to the left of "Late Base" in Table 6.5. And you may find that for a late-

TABLE 6.5. **The Senior Athlete's Seasonal Periods, Their Durations, and Their Training Purposes**

ANNUAL TRAINING PERIOD	PERIOD DURATION	TRAINING PURPOSE	TRAINING DETAILS
Preparation	1–6 weeks	General fitness	Gradually reestablish a structured training routine.
Early Base	3–6 weeks	General fitness	Maximize strength and begin developing aerobic fitness.
Late Base	3–6 weeks	General fitness	Increase high-intensity training and maintain strength.
Build	6–9 weeks	Specific fitness	Train with racelike workouts and maintain strength.
Peak	1–2 weeks	Specific fitness	Taper and simulate small portions of the goal event and maintain strength.
Race	1 week	Specific fitness	Race week. Rest before the event while maintaining race fitness.
Transition	3 days–4 weeks	Rejuvenation	Recover mentally and physically from the stress of serious training.

season A race, you can reestablish your fitness by starting with the Build period. Where you begin training for each of these later-season races depends on how well you've maintained your Base fitness following races earlier in the season. How do you know? Table 6.6 helps answer that question.

Workouts by Period

Table 6.6 suggests the workout priorities for training in each period of the season. All of the workouts in each period are ranked in their order of importance according to the duration of your next A-priority race—

TABLE 6.6. **Priorities of Workout Types According to Race Duration and Seasonal Periods for the Senior Athlete**

	RACE DURATION		
	>4 Hours	**2–4 Hours**	**<2 Hours**
Preparation priorities	1. Aerobic threshold 2. Strength 3. Aerobic capacity	1. Aerobic threshold 2. Strength 3. Aerobic capacity	1. Aerobic threshold 2. Strength 3. Aerobic capacity
Early Base priorities	1. Strength 2. Aerobic threshold 3. Aerobic capacity	1. Strength 2. Aerobic threshold 3. Aerobic capacity	1. Strength 2. Aerobic threshold 3. Aerobic capacity
Late Base priorities	1. Aerobic capacity 2. Aerobic threshold 3. Lactate threshold 4. Strength	1. Lactate threshold 2. Aerobic capacity 3. Aerobic threshold 4. Strength	1. Lactate threshold 2. Aerobic capacity 3. Aerobic threshold 4. Strength
Build priorities	1. Aerobic threshold 2. Lactate threshold 3. Aerobic capacity 4. Strength	1. Lactate threshold 2. Aerobic threshold 3. Aerobic capacity 4. Strength	1. Aerobic capacity 2. Lactate threshold 3. Aerobic threshold 4. Strength
Peak priorities	1. Lactate threshold 2. Strength	1. Lactate threshold 2. Strength	1. Aerobic capacity 2. Strength
Race-week priorities	1. Lactate threshold	1. Lactate threshold	1. Aerobic capacity
Transition priorities	1. Rest and recover	1. Rest and recover	1. Rest and recover

greater than 4 hours, 2 to 4 hours, and less than 2 hours. We can use duration as the determiner since it also controls intensity. The longer the race, the lower the intensity relative to your potential. As the race gets shorter, intensity increases.

The purpose of Table 6.6 is to help you make decisions about the dose of each of the listed workouts by training period. For those workouts ranked as No. 1 in each period, the dose should be the greatest. This workout has the highest priority. It is your key workout each week. The other workouts are also listed in descending order of importance with dosage decreasing as the priority becomes lower.

Let's consider an example of how to use Table 6.6. We'll assume that your next A race is about 3 hours long ("2–4 hours" column), and you are starting the Late Base period. Your highest priority for the week is listed as the lactate-threshold workout. The dose will be the highest for this session, so you may do a total of 36 to 40 minutes of lactate-threshold intervals based on Table 6.1.

The second-highest priority is the aerobic-capacity workout. Since it's a lower-priority workout, you may choose to do a "moderate" dose of 9 to 10 minutes of these intervals. This, again, is taken from Table 6.1.

Third in order of importance for you is the aerobic-threshold workout, so it is assigned a low dose. According to Table 6.1, a low-dose workout for this is 30 minutes to 1 hour long.

The lowest priority is strength training, but by now you should realize that weight lifting at this time in the season is the Strength Maintenance (SM) phase. That's from Table 6.4.

By using these tables, you have laid out an entire week of training in terms of what's most important and the dose for each.

Now that you know how to use Table 6.6, let's return to the question posed previously: How do you know in which period you should start your training for subsequent A-priority races in the season—the second- and, perhaps, third-most-important events you plan to do? The answer has to do with the workouts ranked Numbers 1 and 2 in the late Base period. If after the Transition period following the previous race these seem sound, meaning you've not lost much fitness in these categories, then you will restart your training for the next A-priority race in the

Build period. If you are obviously lacking fitness in these two workout categories, then you should start in the late Base period. If you're not even close to the level of fitness demanded by the late Base period, then your next A-priority race preparation should start in the early Base period, although that's not likely unless you had a very long Transition period after an early-season race.

The "Where do I start training again?" question is never an easy one to answer, as it's based largely on feelings and guesswork. But typically, the longer your taper before the previous A race or the longer the Transition period, the more likely it is that you should start back into training with the late Base period. The shorter period durations, as listed in Table 6.5, should then be long enough to reap the desired fitness benefits for the next A race.

Weekly Routines

So far I've been referring to the shortest training period as a "week." We commonly take that to mean seven days. But when it comes to periodization, that isn't necessarily the case. A week could be any number of days. From this point on, I'll use the term "week" to mean some number of days, not necessarily seven, during which you will do all of the workout types suggested by period in Table 6.6—aerobic-capacity intervals, lactate-threshold intervals, aerobic-threshold steady states, and strength training—along with recovery days.

The reason for changing the duration of a week has to do with density. Seven is the most commonly used number because it fits nicely with a work week. With a seven-day week, shorter workouts can be done Monday through Friday, and longer ones can be done on the weekend, when most athletes have more free time. But seven days may not be optimal for many senior athletes if we consider rate of recovery, physiological capacity for adaptation, and fitness enhancement.

The problem with the seven-day week is that the density may be too great. Trying to shoehorn four demanding workouts into seven days every week may simply be too much for many senior athletes. However, it will definitely work for some who are likely the younger seniors in their 50s. Table 6.7 suggests how a seven-day week may look with all of the key workouts included. Note the high density.

The weekly routine suggested in Table 6.7 may work quite nicely for senior athletes who recover well. The density may be just right. For many others, though, the density is too great and will soon result in excessive fatigue.

This routine may also work for some seniors in the Base period, and certainly in the Preparation period, when training isn't as demanding, but not for the Build period. As the workload increases during the Build period, the density for a seven-day week may prove to be too great. Some seniors, therefore, may be able to use seven days early in the season but need less density in Build. (We'll come back to the Peak and Race periods shortly.)

What should you do if you believe that seven days isn't the best training week for you in one or more periods? The answer is that some number greater than seven must be used. Adding days decreases density by allowing for more recovery days between the hard sessions. It also favors greater doses while ensuring adequate recovery. Table 6.8 suggests a nine-day training week to solve this problem. Note that when we make this change, we can't label the days Monday, Tuesday, and so on because the days on which the key workouts are done will be always changing, but it is easy to incorporate the change into your training plan if you keep a written training diary.

TABLE 6.7. **Suggested Seven-Day Training Routine for Base or Build Period**

DAY	WORKOUT
Monday	Strength training
Tuesday	Aerobic-capacity intervals
Wednesday	Recovery
Thursday	Lactate-threshold intervals
Friday	Strength training or recovery
Saturday	Aerobic-threshold steady state
Sunday	Recovery

As you age and it becomes apparent that you aren't recovering as well as you did when you were a bit younger, you need to make a decision: Either you stick with a seven-day week and cut out a key workout or two, or you change the definition of a "week." The first choice means less fitness, and the second may not be perfect, either. The downside of a nine-day week is that it simply may not fit into your lifestyle. It works best for the senior athlete who is retired or who has a career and lifestyle that are flexible. Career and lifestyle factors may seem trivial as you read this, but the problem will become crystal clear the first time you have to fit a very long aerobic-threshold workout into a day when you also have to be at work by 8 a.m.

There are other ways of designing a training week to match up with your daily routine and your recovery rate. (Remember, your recovery rate may not be the same as that of your training partners, especially if they are significantly younger than you. Respect what your body is telling you, and stick to your plan!) With a little creativity, you may come up with something that works even better for you than seven or nine days. For example, it may be that two recovery days after one of the three hard training sessions in the nine-day week aren't enough. In that case, it may be necessary

TABLE 6.8. **Suggested Nine-Day Training Routine for Base or Build Period**

DAY	WORKOUT
1	Aerobic-capacity intervals
2	Recovery
3	Strength training
4	Lactate-threshold intervals
5	Recovery
6	Strength training or recovery
7	Aerobic-threshold steady state
8	Recovery
9	Recovery

to include three recovery days after each hard day. Your week would then be 12 days long. All of this means that your weekly training routine should be quite flexible; design it to fit your unique needs. Do what best matches your fitness level, recovery schedule, and lifestyle.

Peak and Race Periods

The Peak and Race periods are different from the previous periods and so require special training-week designs. That's because the purpose of training in these periods is no longer increasing fitness but rather producing "form." This term has been used in sport for about a century. It doesn't mean "fitness," as most TV sport commentators imply, but rather "freshness." The purpose of the Peak and Race periods is to have you *fresh* on race day.

Being fresh on race day means being well rested with somewhat high fitness. I say "somewhat" because whenever you increase rest, as you *must* do in these periods to gain form, your fitness declines. Fitness is not increased by resting, although it feels like that is what happens when you rest. What you are sensing is greater freshness that makes it possible for your somewhat reduced fitness to produce your best possible race. The trick is to gain freshness without losing too much fitness. That's done by reducing the duration of workouts and therefore your overall training volume. Fitness is maintained by focusing on intensity.

Training intensity during the Peak and Race periods is determined by your goal race intensity. That intensity goal is likely to be near your aerobic-capacity, lactate-threshold, or aerobic-threshold pace or power; it depends on the duration and type of race you are preparing for. So one of these intensities will become the only one you focus on for key workouts in these last two periods.

The exception is for events lasting longer than 4 hours. A race of 4 hours or longer means that you'll be doing most of the race at or near your aerobic-threshold intensity. Unfortunately, that is too low to maintain fitness, so we'll bump it up a bit in the workouts now. Notice in Table 6.6 that there are only one or two workout types suggested for the Peak and Race periods. In the ">4 Hours" column, the Peak period workouts are "1. Lactate threshold" and "2. Strength." For the same column, the Race period calls for only one workout type, "1. Lactate threshold." At some point during a race that lasts 4 hours or more, it is highly likely that the athlete will approach his or her lactate-threshold intensity. This will probably be on a hill or during a brief stretch into a strong headwind.

Exceptions are any endurance sports that rely heavily on drafting, such as bicycle road racing, wheelchair racing, inline racing, and endurance ice skating. These races are not nearly as steady as, say, running or triathlon; instead, they experience quite variable speeds due to the dynamics of the mass start and the need to draft. So the serious senior athlete in these sports must always stay focused on aerobic-capacity

(VO_2max) intensity in the Build, Peak, and Race periods regardless of the duration of the race.

For the Peak and Race periods for nondrafting races and training, the dual purposes are to increase freshness and to maintain, at as high a level as possible, your fitness. Let's drill down a little deeper into each period to better understand the details.

Peak Period

To increase freshness during the Peak period, the workout durations are gradually shortened, including those for the most intense workouts. This reduction slowly lowers the dosage. The interval workouts may be shortened by doing fewer intervals or by shortening the durations of the intervals. Also during the Peak period, two recovery days follow the interval workouts. This decreases the density of training. By incorporating these changes, freshness will improve while fitness is stabilized. That has the potential to bring you to a peak of readiness by race day.

Table 6.9 provides a suggested routine for planning a two-week Peak period using seven-day weeks, which is the better periodization option now. Note that this may be a one-week period instead of two for any number of reasons having to do with periodization decisions. The most common such situation I've seen is when the athlete was slightly injured or ill and lost a week or so of training during the Build period. In such a situation, Build was extended by one week and Peak shortened to allow for more time to rebuild fitness.

Race Period

The week of the race, called the Race period, has the same purpose as the Peak period: Increase freshness while keeping fitness stable. Now, however, freshness becomes even more critical as race day quickly approaches,

TABLE 6.9. **Example of Seven-Day Training Week in Two-Week Peak Period with Workout Types Based on Expected Race Duration**

	RACE DURATION		
	>4 Hours	2–4 Hours	<2 Hours
Monday	Recovery	Recovery	Recovery
Tuesday	Lactate-threshold intervals	Lactate-threshold intervals	Aerobic-capacity intervals
Wednesday	Strength + recovery	Strength + recovery	Strength + recovery
Thursday	Recovery	Recovery	Recovery
Friday	Lactate-threshold intervals	Lactate-threshold intervals	Aerobic-capacity intervals
Saturday	Recovery	Recovery	Recovery
Sunday	Recovery	Recovery	Recovery
Monday	Lactate-threshold intervals	Lactate-threshold intervals	Aerobic-capacity intervals
Tuesday	Strength + recovery	Strength + recovery	Strength + recovery
Wednesday	Recovery	Recovery	Recovery
Thursday	Lactate-threshold intervals	Lactate-threshold intervals	Aerobic-capacity intervals
Friday	Recovery	Recovery	Recovery
Saturday	Recovery	Recovery	Recovery
Sunday	Lactate-threshold intervals	Lactate-threshold intervals	Aerobic-capacity intervals

so the high-intensity workouts become very short. Each of these includes a warm-up followed by a few intervals before a short cooldown. The intervals are quite short; I always use 90 seconds with the athletes I coach. The recoveries between intervals are relatively long to ensure that fatigue doesn't become a factor in their completion. I use 3 minutes for these. The number of intervals decreases each day so that the total workout time gradually shortens, further reducing both dose and density.

Table 6.10 suggests a race-week routine for further enhancing freshness and race intensity using a seven-day week.

Rest and Test Periods

"Mesocycle" is an important-sounding sports science term for a grouping of similarly purposed training weeks. (Individual weeks are called "microcycles" by scientists.) A mesocycle may encompass several weeks in the Base and Build periods, or it may describe a single week in the Race period. Your training plan will usually call for multiweek mesocycles.

The Base and Build period mesocycles for the senior athlete are usually 14 to 16 days long. For example, if you are doing a nine-day Build period week (see Table 6.6), you would have three such mesocycles—Build 1, Build 2, and Build 3—with each followed by a Rest and Recovery period lasting a few days. You would then test to measure your progress. (This will become clearer when you see examples in "Your Training Plan," which follows.)

Without these R&R breaks at the end of each mesocycle, the likelihood of a breakdown would certainly increase. For the senior athlete, R&R may last three to five days. During that time, all workouts are short and easy. "Short" is a relative term. For an athlete who trains 14 hours per week, short may mean 1 hour, whereas for someone whose weekly volume is

TABLE 6.10. **Example of Seven-Day Training Week in Race Week Based on Expected Race Duration**

	RACE DURATION		
	>4 Hours	2–4 Hours	<2 Hours
Monday	Recovery	Recovery	Recovery
Tuesday	5 × 90 sec at lactate threshold (3-min recoveries)	5 × 90 sec at lactate threshold (3-min recoveries)	5 × 90 sec at aerobic capacity (3-min recoveries)
Wednesday	4 × 90 sec at lactate threshold (3-min recoveries)	4 × 90 sec at lactate threshold (3-min recoveries)	4 × 90 sec at aerobic capacity (3-min recoveries)
Thursday	3 × 90 sec at lactate threshold (3-min recoveries)	3 × 90 sec at lactate threshold (3-min recoveries)	3 × 90 sec at aerobic capacity (3-min recoveries)
Friday	Recovery or day off	Recovery or day off	Recovery or day off
Saturday	2 × 90 sec at lactate threshold (3-min recoveries)	2 × 90 sec at lactate threshold (3-min recoveries)	2 × 90 sec at aerobic capacity (3-min recoveries)
Sunday	Race	Race	Race

7 hours, short may be 30 minutes. "Easy" is, well, easier to define. It's always going to be zone 1 whether you are using a heart rate monitor, a speed-and-distance device, or a power meter (see Appendix C).

Three days are about right for the senior athlete who recovers fairly quickly and is using a training week that provides a proper density. For the senior who recovers more slowly or who has been training with very high density, four or five days of R&R is better. How do you know which R&R duration is best for you? When you find yourself feeling fresh and champing at the bit to train harder, it's time move on to the next activity—testing.

The first day after the R&R break in the Base and Build periods is a good time to test your progress, since you are well rested. The test may be done in a lab or other such testing facility that you use consistently. Using different test locations could result in widely divergent data, so I recommend that you always remain consistent with testing.

The same goes for field tests: Stay consistent. The procedures for aerobic-capacity, lactate-threshold, and aerobic-threshold field tests are described in Appendix B, "Field Tests for Senior Athletes." Select the field test that matches your unique workout priority No. 1 from Table 6.6. Again, be consistent by using the same course for your test every time. Do your best to keep the other variables as similar as possible from one test to the next. This includes time of day, eating prior to the test, equipment selection, and anything else that may be unique to your sport.

The day after the test is a recovery day again. On the following day, training resumes with the next mesocycle.

These Test and Rest periods are also good times to do B-priority races. B-priority races are those that are important for you but not as important as the A races, and they are excellent for gauging your progress in the sort of situations for which you are actually training. Scheduling them at the end of an R&R break means you will be fairly fresh going into them and should get good results. The other type of race is the C-priority. These are the least important races, which you are doing only to get a hard workout. When they occur in your training schedule is unimportant. The results are also not important.

Table 6.11 lays out a suggested Rest and Test period based on a seven-day week with five days of Rest and Recovery followed by a test and then another day of rest. Seven days works best for R&R plus testing. Your schedule could even be shorter than seven days if you need only three or four days of R&R before testing. It's also possible that you won't always

TABLE 6.11. **Example of a Five-Day Rest and Recovery Break and a Two-Day Rest and Test Period Following a 13-, 14-, or 16-Day Base and Build Mesocycle**

DAY	WORKOUT
1	Short and easy recovery workout or day off
2	Short and easy recovery workout
3	Short and easy recovery workout
4	Short and easy recovery workout
5	Short and easy recovery workout
6	Test
7	Short and easy recovery workout or day off

feel the need to test after every Base and Build mesocycle. So your next mesocycle could start as soon as R&R ends or after the two-day Test and Rest period.

Note that if you are planning to use a nine-day week in either the Base or Build periods, the last two days are always recovery days (see Table 6.8). Those two days at the end of the second week may instead be considered the first two days of your R&R. There is no reason to take two days of recovery followed by three to five days of R&R; just merge them. This makes the duration of such a mesocycle 16 days (9 + 7) instead of 18. In the same way, if you train with a seven-day week and the last day is always for recovery, you can merge it in with the R&R break. That makes that last week of such a mesocycle six days instead of seven.

Your Training Plan

Whew! I've thrown a lot of periodization details at you in this chapter. I expect you may be feeling somewhat overwhelmed. Your head is probably spinning. You may even be persuaded to just forget about all of this planning stuff and go back to working out as you've been doing. Don't give up. The sport-science-y stuff you've been reading about in this chapter has the potential to greatly improve your performance. And while it may seem complex so far, in this section I'm going to return to the real world of training. By the time you finish this section, you can have a plan that closely matches your needs and produces fast racing. Hang in there just a bit longer!

Before getting started on your training plan, let's take a look at two examples of how it can be done. Figure 6.1 shows how you might prepare for the first A-priority race of the season using seven-day weeks. Figure 6.2 does the same based on nine-day weeks in the Base and Build periods. These two examples assume it's midwinter and you are starting to think about your first race of the coming season. If you are already into the race season and beyond your first A-priority race, you will start your plan with either a Late Base period or a Build period. In that case, your mesocycles will likely be shorter than what is suggested in these examples since your fitness is already fairly high from the previous several months of training. It doesn't take as much time to maintain fitness as to initially develop it. Table 6.5 lists the possible duration ranges for each period.

Let's take a closer look at these examples. Both assume that the first A-priority race of the season is on Sunday, July 12, and they both start the training season preparing for it on the previous December 29. Also the same is everything from June 15 through July 19. That includes the last R&R, the last Test and Rest period, Peak 1, Peak 2, Race week, and the Transition period. That's quite a bit, but it's as far as the similarity goes. Everything else is scheduled differently.

On close examination, you will notice that the Preparation period is five weeks long in Figure 6.1 but only about two in Figure 6.2. Table 6.5 suggests that it may be one to six weeks. The Preparation period steps up

FIGURE 6.1. **Calendar example with 7-day weeks for every period**

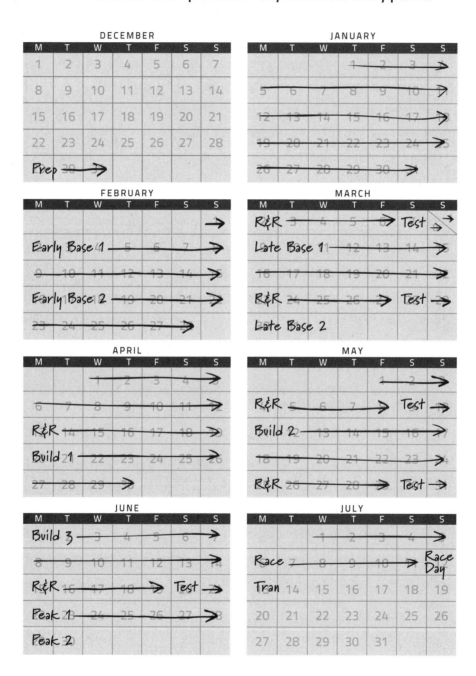

FIGURE 6.2. **Calendar example using both 7-day (Preparation, Peak, Race, Transition) and 9-day weeks (Base, Build)**

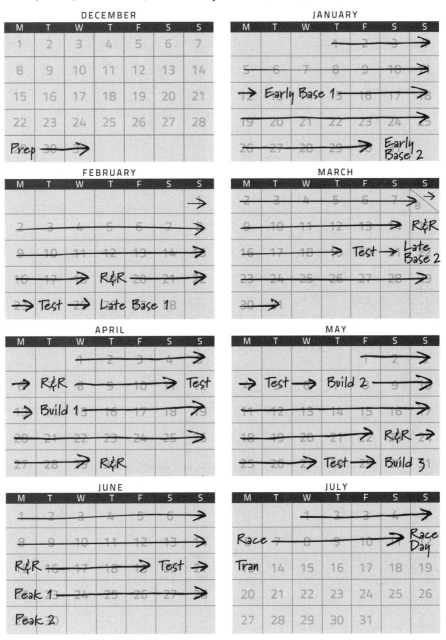

the seriousness of your training only slightly. For the serious senior athlete, it is defined by light training in three training domains: aerobic threshold, strength, and aerobic capacity (see Table 6.6). The reason for the fairly broad duration range is that the only purpose of this period is to gradually reestablish a structured training routine. You may well be able to accomplish that objective in a few days and not need a long period. Then again, you may enjoy a long, easygoing transition to serious training as you come back from your previous season's rejuvenation break in the Transition period. That may have been as much as a month during which time you didn't "train" but rather "played" whenever and however you wanted. It was pretty laid back. There was no purpose other than to rest, recover, rejuvenate, and enjoy life.

Note that there is no R&R break in the Early Base 1 period in both figures. In that stage of the training year, the dose and density of training are both fairly low, so Early Base 1 and Early Base 2 blend together in an unbroken string of several weeks. If you will otherwise train using a nine-day week, you may consider instead following a seven-day weekly platform in these Early Base periods since the training is not very stressful. Of course, if at any time you do feel the need for a few days of rest, don't hesitate to take an R&R break.

The first R&R and Test and Rest periods come at the end of Early Base 2. This is the time to make sure you are rested before starting the more serious training of Late Base. The testing is done now to establish a baseline for your fitness and also to make sure that your training zones are set correctly. To set your training zones, perform the lactate-threshold test as described in Appendix B. Depending on your race duration, you may also want to test aerobic capacity (race duration less than 2 hours) or aerobic threshold (race duration greater than 4 hours). These tests are also explained in Appendix B.

Returning to Figure 6.1, note that each of the training periods (Early Base, Late Base, Build, Peak, Race, and Transition) starts on a Monday. What produces that pattern is the length of the R&R periods. You may recall that these are typically three to five days long. In Figure 6.1, the athlete chose five days every time. This would be common for an athlete who recovers slowly and needs the maximum time possible to bounce back and get ready for the two-day Test and Rest period. Combining a five-day R&R with a two-day Test and Rest makes for a seven-day period at the end of Early Base 2, Late Base 1 and 2, and each of the Build periods.

Had the athlete chosen to schedule three- or four-day R&R breaks followed by the standard two-day Test and Rest period, the start of the following period would have occurred on Saturday or Sunday. That obviously means the following Base and Build periods would no longer begin on a Monday. The weekly schedule would then become similar to the nine-day weekly platform, in which the critical workouts don't always occur on the same day of the week. Such a pattern could really mess up how your training and lifestyle blend together, which is the main reason for choosing the seven-day training week. One way to avoid this conundrum is to lengthen the first week of the mesocycle following a combined R&R plus Rest and Test of five or six days. For example, if you plan for a four-day R&R plus two-day Rest and Test each time, you could start the next week on Sunday instead of Monday. That would make this week eight days long. The "extra" workout inserted on that first Sunday could be a long recovery session or an aerobic-threshold workout, keeping in mind that on Monday you have a strength session and on Tuesday aerobic-capacity intervals (see Table 6.7). In other words, this first training day shouldn't be highly stressful.

Note that both Figures 6.1 and 6.2 have the first A-priority race of the season planned for a Sunday. If it is instead on a Saturday, the week of the Race period should be shortened to six days with each of the workouts

(Table 6.10) moved back one day. It may be necessary to make that Monday a rest day if the preceding Sunday was a high-dose workout.

Given these examples and all of the tables and discussion about them in this chapter, you should now be able to come up with a good overall training plan for your season. All you need is a calendar—either a standard paper calendar or an electronic calendar, whichever you are more comfortable using. If it's paper, be sure to write your plan in pencil, as there will likely be changes.

Start your calendar by listing your next A-priority race on the date it occurs. Then work backward, using the period durations from Table 6.5 and Figures 6.1 and 6.2 as guides to determine when your Race, Peak 2, Peak 1, Build 3, Build 2, Build 1, Late Base 2, Late Base 1, Early Base 2, Early Base 1, and Preparation periods will start.

Insert a Transition period starting the day after the race. This period follows the first and second A-priority races of the season. For Transition, you should include a few days to a full week (or perhaps more) of Rest and Recovery. After the last race of the season, which may be your second or third A-priority race, this period could be as much as four weeks long. That's common after a very demanding season of training that leaves you deeply fatigued both physically and mentally.

Once you have a finished plan on paper (or on an electronic device), the tricky part is where the rubber meets the road—applying it. It's critical that you are flexible in following the plan. What does "flexible" mean? It means paying close attention to how you feel every day. If you are not feeling rested enough to do a high-dose workout, even though one may be planned for that day, you must reduce its dose—the intensity, the duration, or both. Even consider taking the day off if your fatigue is great enough. Training through deep fatigue will result only in a poor-quality session and more fatigue, not better fitness.

Planning your season's periodization is only a tool to help you train more effectively. Too many see it as a rigid dictum requiring you to do every workout as scheduled regardless of how you feel at the time. Tackling it so rigidly is a sure way to end up ill, injured, or overtrained.

There are a few athletes—and I do mean "few"—who are so in tune with their bodies and have such a depth of experience with training that they don't need detailed and written training plans. You may know of good athletes like this who express disdain for periodization and planning. Yet they do good workouts, recover well, and have great races. Regardless of what they may say, however, they *do* have a plan. And they *are* periodizing. It just isn't written down and worked out in detail on a daily and seasonal basis, as I've suggested. It's in their heads. They know what needs to be done and when. Dose and density are always on their minds even if they don't know what the terms mean. What they're doing is called "periodization on demand" and "recovery on demand," which work well for a small number of athletes.

Most athletes, however, are incapable of training this way because they give only lip service to "listening to their bodies." In reality, many who scorn periodization and planning follow the philosophy of "never enough." That approach almost always results in serious breakdowns.

Once your plan is complete you must assume that it will change as you start using it. In more than 30 years of coaching athletes, I've never had anyone complete a season with their original plan unchanged. Things happen. You catch a cold and miss a few workouts. You get busy in your job, causing you to miss several training sessions. Or something else gets in the way. I know you understand this because it happens to all of us from time to time. When interruptions happen, you need to give some thought as to how you might revise the training plan going forward.

If you missed three or fewer days of training, just continue on as if it never happened.

If you missed four to seven days, consider it an R&R period and reschedule going forward. And consider omitting Peak 1 in order to re-establish a higher fitness level before tapering.

If you missed more than a week, it is probably a good idea to take a step back one full period to rebuild your previous fitness.

If you missed more than two weeks of training, it's usually best to return to Late Base 2 followed by Build 1. You may have to omit the last few weeks of the Build period in this situation. In this case, it will take a lot of head scratching to come up with a revised plan. Just bear in mind that the Base period has a higher priority than the more advanced Build period whenever fitness is lost. And it's usually a good idea when such a training catastrophe happens to leave out Peak 1 to allow for more fitness to be developed before tapering.

The most useful advice I can give for any lost-training situation is that you should not try to make up the missed workouts by piling them on top of the remaining sessions on your schedule.

Advanced Training

The purpose of this chapter was to answer the question "When should I do the high-dose workouts described in the previous chapters?" This seemingly simple query raises many issues such as how great the key workout doses should be and how densely they should be spaced. The density question also raises the matter of how many days to include in a week. There I suggested that a good alternative for the serious senior athlete is to train in nine-day "weeks." Nine days allow for more recovery between high-dose workouts, thus lowering the density of training. Density is the critical concern of the serious senior athlete.

That's a lot of details to answer what seems like a simple question. But there were even more details needed to do it right, such as how to taper for an A-priority race and how and when to test progress toward your race-fitness goal.

All of these details brought us to the conclusion that a plan is necessary if you are to race fast and perform at a high level as a competitor. By using the many planning tables in this chapter and following the examples of training plans provided (Figures 6.1 and 6.2), you should now have a detailed plan for your next race.

Creating such a seasonal plan is much like preparing for a long cross-country drive. It's a rare person who would take such a journey without a map and a travel plan. Even with a travel plan, you can expect changes along the way, such as detours for construction or better routes that become obvious as you go. You should expect the same for your training plan. The obstacles will be things that pop up in your life unexpectedly, such as illness, work-related projects, or family matters. These things happen to even the best athletes. Be ready for them by being flexible with how you travel down the planned route to your race. It's okay to miss workouts from time to time in order to get rested. It's perfectly fine to rearrange the weekly training plan in order to accommodate the unexpected in your life.

The glaring omission from this chapter was what to do on recovery days and in the R&R breaks. These are some of the most critical times for the senior athlete who frequently trains with high-dose workouts. This topic is so important that I decided to devote an entire chapter to it. That's where we're headed next.

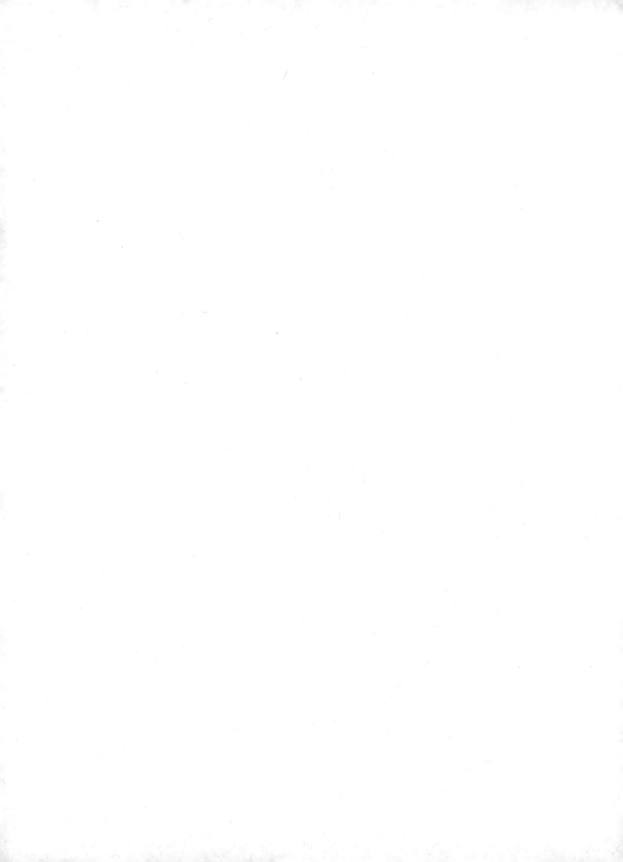

REST AND RECOVERY

We don't stop playing because we grow old.
We grow old because we stop playing.

—GEORGE BERNARD SHAW

When I was in college in the 1960s, I was a runner on the track team. The coach used to have us do a standard workout several times each week. It was similar to what I've been calling aerobic-capacity intervals. Back then, though, I called this workout "intervals 'til you puke."

We'd warm up on our own, and then the coach would blow his whistle. That meant we were to jog over to where he was sitting in the stands next to the start-finish line on the track. He looked a bit like a big-bellied Buddha holding a stopwatch and can of Coke. We knew what was next: 440-yard intervals (we didn't have metric tracks back then). We never knew how many intervals we were going to do or how fast we should run them other than "as fast as possible." We didn't know how to pace them or how long the recoveries would be. We might do a dozen or 15 or 7. Nobody knew—not even the coach. When one of us eventually threw up after a few such intervals, our coach would give us a longer recovery and we'd do only a few more of the dreaded intervals. We always hoped that someone would toss his cookies so we could get it over with. The cookie tosser was often me. That was sports science 50 years ago.

The amazing thing was, at age 20 I could do that workout five days in a row with only two days of recovery in a week (no one trained on the weekends back then). Today if I tried to do five aerobic-capacity interval workouts ('til I puked!) in a single week, I'd soon be wasted. By the third back-to-back day of those workouts, my performance would be rapidly going south. The fourth or fifth such session (if I managed to even start them) would be a joke. I simply cannot recover nearly as quickly these days.

I hear the same thing about recovery from nearly all the serious senior athletes whom I talk with about getting older. We all agree that we recover more slowly. But is it a fact that recovery takes longer as we age? Well, there is at least one interesting study on this topic. A few years ago, some Australian sports scientists compared the recovery perceptions of nine older cyclists with those of nine younger ones.[1] All were well trained. Each of the 18 subjects did three consecutive days of 30-minute time trials and reported their subjective measures of soreness, fatigue, and recovery every day. While there were no big swings in performance over the three days for either group, the older athletes reported significantly higher levels of soreness and fatigue and lower levels of recovery. From such limited research on this topic, scientists have concluded that the muscles of folks our age are more susceptible to damage from intense exercise, that we have a slower repair process, and that our adaptation response ("super-compensation") isn't as effective as it is in younger athletes.[2]

That single paper doesn't give us much to go on regarding the vagaries of recovery in aging athletes, but based on what I've experienced and what older athletes tell me, it seems right on. It also seems that getting everything just right in our lifestyles is increasingly critical to our recovery.

The two most important recovery components are sleep and nutrition. Of course that's true for all athletes, regardless of age. When you are young, though, you can mess these up quite a bit and get away with it. In college I'd often stay up most of the night studying and eating crappy food, and yet I'd manage to do puke intervals several times a week with little degradation in performance. Not anymore. These days, I try to leave nothing to chance when it comes to recovery. It's a good thing that wisdom comes with growing older because we have to be wise to keep up with all the physical vicissitudes of advancing age.

Not only does slow recovery cause a reduction in the density of training, it also increases the risk of injury. As older athletes, we are more susceptible to joint, tendon, and muscle damage, and once the soreness sets in, we heal more slowly than young athletes do.[3] That's a double whammy for our performance.

Despite all of this, many athletes do nothing to enhance their recovery. A 2013 study of 212 veteran cyclists over the age of 35, both male and female, found that 47 percent did not have any recovery strategy after workouts or races.[4] They apparently just let nature run its course while hoping for the best. For those who did have a recovery plan, the most common method was stretching, which has little value for enhancing recovery.[5] Of course, having no recovery strategy may have been more prevalent with the young vets than with the seniors in the study. We don't know as there has been no such research done only on us oldsters.

Fatigue Markers

You could not have made it this far in sport without understanding that workouts must be both hard and easy. In the context of training for endurance sport, "hard" means long duration or high intensity—high dose.

When it comes to high dose, the key for the serious and experienced athlete is intensity. That's why I've proposed that high-intensity training is the key to your performance improvement after age 50 (and for many years to come). Fast intervals and heavy strength-building loads play a major role in achieving such a lofty goal.

Hard workouts require recovery, of course, and several times in previous chapters I've suggested that you must pay attention to your recovery from workouts. However, I have not spelled out the details. So how much recovery do you need, and how frequently should you recover? While there is no precise formula to determine when you need to take a break and how long it should be, we do have general guidelines, described in Chapter 6, that are based on markers of fatigue. These markers will tell you when to back off. They are indicators that you are tired, and although none are rock-solid indicators that tell you without any doubt that it's time to recover, you know that recovery is incomplete as long as any of these markers are present.

Of course, you'll never shed 100 percent of your fatigue with only a day or two of recovery between hard sessions. It takes several days, as in a multiday Rest and Recovery break, to become fully rested. Keep in mind as you review the following common indicators that you are experiencing some degree of normal fatigue.

Perceived Fatigue

Perceived fatigue is the most basic and common way to gauge the need for recovery. It's as simple as asking, "How do I feel?" You must be honest in answering. Common subjective signs that you are fatigued include muscle soreness, unusually poor sleep, low motivation to exercise, general malaise, localized leg or arm fatigue, heavier-than-normal breathing during easy workouts, and unusual difficulty in walking up a flight of stairs.

Mood

Your mood may also be a good predictor of your fatigue.[6] When you're moody, the fun is gone from life. Grumpiness is my best indicator. I know I need more rest when I find myself becoming angry at stoplights. Sometimes those closest to you know when you're in need of recovery, as you're not your normal happy self. Pay close attention to how you interact with the world around you. If you're moody, that's a pretty good sign that fatigue is present and that you need to back off on your workouts and get some rest.

Waking Heart Rate

Although not thoroughly researched, change in waking heart rate has been used for decades by athletes to determine their state of fatigue.[7] Of course, to use this method effectively you must first know your baseline waking heart rate, so check and record your heart rate on waking near the end of a multiday Rest and Recovery break. This will give you the baseline number. Then, during your standard training weeks, check your waking pulse daily, before you get out of bed and while still lying down, to see how it compares. You may find, as many do, that it is elevated 10 percent or more above the baseline when you also have other signs of fatigue such as muscle soreness or moodiness. If so, you need to rest and recover before your next hard training block.

Heart Rate Variability

Heart rate variability (HRV) is a newcomer to fatigue-recovery determination.[8] When someone is well rested, the interval between heartbeats at rest varies. When an athlete is fatigued, though, the length of these between-heartbeat intervals remains relatively constant. Currently, the equipment necessary to measure HRV is rather expensive, but expect to see some less-costly options in the near future. One such device currently in the early stages of development is a smartphone app used in combination with a standard heart rate monitor. This technique has a lot of potential.

Physical Signs

You may notice other physical signs that you need more rest, such as itchy eyes, a runny nose, or the appearance of cold sores on your lips. Paying attention to such seemingly little things can help you become wiser and better at determining your state of fatigue.

• • •

When any of the preceding indicators are present, use sleep and nutrition as your primary tools to fully reap the performance benefits of recovery from hard training. You've got to dial in both of them if you're going to recover quickly and train well—they can't be left to chance. There are other things you can add to your recovery plan, and later in this chapter we'll examine the methods that may help to enhance your recuperation between high-dose workouts and during extended R&R breaks from training. But they are secondary to sleep and nutrition. So let's start with the two most important enhancers of recovery—snoozing and eating.

Sleep and Recovery

The purpose of sleep is the growth and rejuvenation of the body: the muscular, skeletal, immune, nervous, and other systems. Sleep is your primary means of recovery from training stress. There is nothing else you can do that will help you recover faster or more completely. Sleep is critical to sport success and not something to mess around with, yet many choose to shorten their sleep time in order to pack more stuff into their lives. It's quite common for athletes to stay up late watching their favorite TV shows and then set an alarm so they can get up early the next morning in order to fit in a workout before heading off to work. If you depend on an alarm clock to wake you, then you probably aren't getting enough sleep—or enough recovery. Going to bed earlier would more than likely improve your performance. That single lifestyle change may even improve your life in other ways.

Several studies have found that the amount of sleep you get is closely associated with not only your health but also your longevity. Short sleep durations have been shown to increase the risk of obesity, heart disease, and type 2 diabetes.[9] Conversely, those who report regularly sleeping six to seven hours per night appear to have long life spans.[10] Interestingly, sleeping more than seven hours nightly has been associated, at least in one study, with a shorter life.[11] Note that "association" doesn't mean "cause" but simply correlation, meaning only that the two were found to occur together. There *could* be a cause-and-effect connection, but it isn't known with any degree of certainty. Even if long sleep were causal, it shouldn't be taken to mean that setting an alarm to wake you up after seven hours in bed is the key to a long life. A naturally occurring sleep duration is probably best for longevity as well as health. Your normal nightly sleep duration is probably determined by genetics[12] and shouldn't be artificially shortened. It is probably beneficial to wake up naturally rather than to the buzzing of a clock.

To appreciate the benefits of sleep for recovery it's helpful to understand sleep. What happens during slumber that produces renewal so that you can do another hard workout? Let's start by finding out what goes on in your body when you're asleep.

Sleep researchers divide your snooze time into two broad periods called rapid eye movement (REM) and non–rapid eye movement (NREM).[13]

NREM is further divided into three stages—N1, N2, and N3. The last of these is referred to as "slow-wave sleep" because the frequency of the brain's electrical activity becomes quite low. In a full night of normal sleep, your body progresses through the N1, N2, N3, and REM stages several times. Slow-wave sleep makes up much of the early stages of a full night of sleep, with most of the REM time occurring in the latter half of the night. These two stages have a lot to do with how well you recover, so let's take a closer look at them.

Sleep Stages

Your body operates on a built-in clock called the "circadian rhythm." This clock is set by how much light enters your eyes. In the evening, around sunset, your clock initiates the release of the hormone melatonin from the pineal gland in the brain. Your brain lowers your body temperature at the same time. This produces the drowsiness and yawning that is the start of the N1 stage. As with most hormones, melatonin production decreases as you get older.[14] This implies that sleepiness for some oldsters may not be as compelling as it is for younger athletes. Yet many older athletes find that they become drowsy much earlier in the evening than they did when young and may even fall asleep in a chair long before making it to the bedroom. These older athletes also tend to wake up earlier in the morning.[15]

Older athletes also frequently experience insomnia due to a circadian clock that is out of rhythm. This is especially common for women who are entering menopause and for some who are postmenopausal. A review of the scientific research of 12,603 women of various ethnicities at this stage of life found that 38 percent of them had difficulty sleeping.[16] Most of the sleeplessness was reported by women who were in the early stages of menopause—"perimenopause." This transition stage may last four to eight years. Caucasian women appear to have more sleep disturbances than other ethnic groups, with Asians having the least. The lifestyle difficulties of menopause are something that should be discussed with your physician.

Getting back to melatonin, a specific type of light, called "blue light," which is produced by the sun, interferes with its production. The light-bulbs in your home also give off some blue light—not nearly as much as the sun but possibly enough to hinder melatonin release. To help stimulate melatonin in order to start feeling drowsy, you can turn off most of the lights before bedtime. There are also special blue-blocking glasses that look like sunglasses and can be worn in the evening if you must be in a bright, artificially lit room.[17] Search the Internet to find such products.

Sleep Stages and Hormones

While there is still a lot to be learned about sleep, it appears that each stage has a specific, essential purpose. The two with which we are most concerned are the REM and slow-wave (N3) stages. Those are when most of your recovery occurs.

REM is the truly high-quality stage of sleep, when most recovery happens. REM is also when you do most of your memorable dreaming. This stage lasts for a few minutes at a time and makes up 20 to 25 percent of your sleep time if you have a full night of sleep. REM happens about every 90 minutes to 2 hours, with NREM or brief awakenings making up the in-between times. During REM the tissue-building hormones testosterone and estrogen are released into the body to aid recovery. These hormones are categorized as anabolic steroids, meaning that they promote growth and repair of muscles and bones. They also have a positive effect on other cellular properties that improve endurance performance; for example, they help build the capillary network for blood delivery to the muscles.

In terms of recovery, testosterone is the more potent of these two hormones. Figure 7.1 shows what happens to the testosterone levels of men[18] and women as they age (data are lacking on testosterone in women relative to age, so this figure relies on a rough estimate). Men produce about 20 times as much testosterone as women, but women's bodies are more sensitive to it. Since REM occurs late in a night's sleep cycle, artificially shortening your sleep by awakening to an alarm clock may well diminish the release of these hormones, thus hindering full recovery.[19] The negative

FIGURE 7.1. **Changes in total free testosterone in men and women with aging**

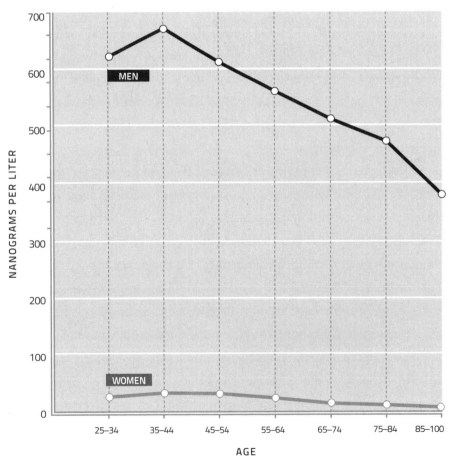

FIGURE 7.2. **Decline of growth hormone with aging**

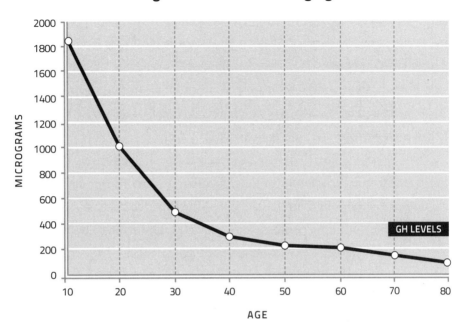

results may not be too great after a night or two of lost REM time, but chronically shortening your natural sleep cycle is likely to have a long-term effect on training quality and performance.

The other critical recovery sleep stage is slow wave (N3). It generally starts about an hour after falling asleep and recurs several times during the first half or so of the night. During this time your body experiences a rush of growth hormone (GH) that promotes muscle growth and bone repair. Nearly half of your daily GH secretion occurs during this stage.[20] That's why pro athletes often take naps—they're trying to increase their GH production. Short of losing an entire night of sleep, you're unlikely to miss your daily dose of growth hormone. But since aging reduces the total amount of growth hormone your body produces, you can't afford to miss any sleep at all.[21] Figure 7.2 illustrates what happens to GH with aging.

Unfortunately, slow-wave sleep duration is shortened in older folks, as we tend to wake up more often.[22] In college-aged youth, slow-wave sleep makes up about 19 percent of sleep time. For us old folks, it's more like 3 percent.[23] That makes for a huge reduction in recovery-enhancing GH. Combine that with reduced testosterone production due to low-quality REM sleep and using an alarm clock to wake up, and it's no wonder your fitness and performance are going south.

Overall, with aging there is a tendency for an earlier onset of sleep in the evening, an earlier morning awakening, and more-fragmented and shallower sleep throughout the night. This further decreases the release of the anabolic hormones testosterone and GH. Unfortunately, cortisol,[24] another hormone largely unchanged with age, is released into the bloodstream while we sleep. Cortisol's primary function is to prepare the body to cope with stress by increasing blood sugar (we'll investigate the downsides of this in Chapter 8) while also compromising the immune system. It's also been shown to slow the healing of injuries[25] and decrease bone formation.[26]

Improving Your Sleep

Despite the double whammy of the hormone issues, sleep is very definitely the key to better performance with aging. To help maximize sleep time, there are a few things you can do that may prove beneficial besides wearing blue-blocking glasses in the evening, which may make you feel a bit weird. I expect you are already familiar with the most common ones—avoiding caffeine in the late afternoon, not working out intensely in the four hours or so before bedtime, maintaining a calm and quiet environment before going to bed, following a regular sleep schedule, and bedding down in a dark and cool room. These are all good practices, and there are others as well.

Go light on alcohol in the evening, as it has a rebound effect that can wake you later from an otherwise sound sleep. While alcohol doesn't seem to negatively affect slow-wave sleep and may even be beneficial for it, it has been shown to reduce REM sleep duration.[27]

Some athletes take a melatonin supplement in the evening to promote drowsiness. I don't recommend it because typically when a supplement is used exogenously ("from outside the body") to promote some functional change, the body responds by reducing or even halting its natural production of the targeted product while possibly becoming less sensitive to it. An alternative solution that some studies have reported is drinking a glass of tart cherry juice in the evening. I know that sounds strange, but it seems to work. The aging subjects in these cherry-juice studies had an increase in melatonin production and improved sleep compared with a placebo.[28] Again, weird—but possibly beneficial.

The hour when you eat your evening meal and what it is made up of may also affect your nighttime sleeping. As your mom told you when you were a kid (of course, you didn't pay any attention), a late-evening meal or large prebedtime snack can reduce sleep quality, so don't chow down right before going to bed.[29] One study—*only* one so far, and one that has great room for improvement—has shown that the foods you eat late in the day may affect how well you sleep.[30] University of North Dakota researchers looked at which types of food were most likely to improve your sleep and, conversely, which may have negative consequences. Forty-four adult subjects ate either a high-protein, a high-fat, a high-carbohydrate, or a balanced control diet before retiring for the evening. They did this over a four-day period and crossed over so that each subject ate all of the four meal types. They went to bed at a regular time after each of the meals, and their sleep quality was measured. The fewest sleep interruptions came after the high-protein meal. The high-carb meals produced the least-restful sleep. So the bottom line is that it may be advantageous for your subsequent sleep, especially if you typically don't sleep well, to eat a little additional protein rather than more carbohydrate for supper or a prebedtime snack.

I want to once again emphasize that sleep is the single most important thing you can do to speed your recovery. It will complement your high-quality training while helping you avoid setbacks due to injury, illness, and overtraining. If you artificially shorten your sleep by using an alarm clock to wake up, then you simply aren't snoozing enough. If you don't sleep well—meaning that your sleep is interrupted by long periods of being awake—or you don't sleep at least six hours per night, then you need to take corrective steps. Without adequate sleep, anything else that you do in training will have a greatly reduced benefit simply because your recovery will always be lacking.

Nutrition and Recovery

The second-most-important component of recovery is nutrition. Over the past 20 years of my life, between ages 50 and 70, I've made some significant changes to my diet. Until I was 50, though, I ate much the same diet during and after college. As I look back, I'm appalled by all of the junk food in my daily diet—cookies, potato chips, pastries, soft drinks, and more. The list is almost endless. I suppose I was just being a typical young American male. Yet despite the poor average quality of my diet, I still managed to train and race well. Could I have been a better athlete? Possibly, although there is something about being young that allows us to get away with a lot of dietary mistakes. I've watched my son, Dirk, go through the same process as a road cyclist. Now that he's in his mid-40s, he is beginning to make adjustments to his diet in order to perform better after 30 years of top-level racing. He's fixing his diet at a younger age than I did, and he'll probably benefit from the change sooner than I did, too.

While what you eat is important to recovery, whatever foods and eating patterns you find work well for you shouldn't be compromised as you get older as long as you are getting good results. If you are seeing a decline in performance, though, you should look at your diet. A diet based largely on junk food will catch up with you at some point in the aging process. It's not a matter of if but rather when.

I expect you've already discovered that food quality has something to do with your recovery and performance. By age 50 it's generally becoming apparent to most. Only a few, truly unique aging athletes can continue eating lots of junk food and still perform at a high level well into their 50s, 60s, and 70s. Most certainly cannot.

But simply eliminating junk food isn't the full story. If one source of energy is eliminated, some other source must take its place. So what should you eat more of after cutting out the junk? And of nearly equal importance, when should you eat it? If you haven't discovered what foods and eating patterns work best for your recovery and training, then you may get some ideas in this section. Chapter 8 will examine the topic of diet in much greater detail.

Recovery and Your Chronic Diet

The two most common diets chosen by endurance athletes are high-carbohydrate and high-fat diets. By "high" I mean a chronic (daily) diet in which at least half of one's calories come from either carbs or fat. High-protein diets are rare, but protein plays an important and unique role in the recovery of senior athletes, so we'll examine that macronutrient in a separate section.

Our purpose is not to take your chronic diet in a new direction but rather to better understand how you can eat to speed recovery. We'll do that by examining the types of foods you can choose at various times in order to produce the fastest and most complete recovery for you given the normal diet that you already eat. In the next chapter we'll more thoroughly examine diet in terms of what may be the best chronic diet for you as an aging athlete. In this section, though, we're thinking only in terms of eating for recovery from exercise.

As mentioned, the chronic diets we are considering are those made up primarily of either carbohydrate or fat. For most athletes, a high-fat diet is hard to comprehend because it doesn't follow the normal set of nutritional "rules" for exercise and recovery. For example, the primary rule that most athletes accept at face value is that fuel must be frequently ingested during long exercise and in the hours afterward in order to produce movement and physical recovery. Another rule is that the tank must be topped off before starting to exercise. But the high-fat diet doesn't follow these rules. How can that be?

The starting point for understanding the high-fat diet is that the body has different sources of fuel that it can call on to produce energy. The two most common sources are carbohydrate and fat. (Protein is also a potential fuel source but is used in comparatively minute amounts.) Without going into all of the physiology behind the fueling of exercise, we'll condense the explanation to say that when eating the typical high-carb diet, the body relies heavily on glucose, a sugar, for fuel. Even when the tank is full, glucose is quite limited in the athlete's body; depending on body size, high-carb athletes store around 1,500 to 2,000 calories of glucose in their bodies (most of it in the muscles). That's enough to last perhaps 2 to 3 hours at a duration-specific, high-intensity effort. So fuel must be ingested before starting exercise in order to top off the limited levels. More fuel must be taken in during exercise to keep the muscles functioning, and carbohydrate also needs to be replaced soon after exercise to restock the depleted tank. These are the rules that most endurance athletes are used to following. The

Eating for Recovery on a High-Carb Diet

When following a high-carb diet, it's necessary to take in carbohydrate frequently in order to perform and recover well. Each high-dose workout has feeding times linked with it. I call these "stages." Here's how they work.

STAGE 1 Before the workout

The goal of this stage is to have adequate carbohydrate stored in order to get you comfortably through the first 90 minutes of the workout. For workouts shorter than an hour, don't sweat it. For longer morning sessions, though, prefueling is especially important. Eating 200 to 400 calories primarily from a moderate-glycemic-index, carbohydrate-rich food (for example, fruit or oatmeal) two hours before the workout would be perfect, but that often isn't possible. Few are willing to get up at 3 a.m. just to eat before a 5 a.m. session on a workday. As an alternative for these early-morning sessions, 10 minutes before the workout begins, start taking in a bottle of your favorite sports drink or a couple of gel packets with 12 ounces of water. That's your "breakfast." This isn't quite as good as eating a real breakfast two hours before but far better than training on a low fuel tank.

STAGE 2 During the workout

Now you need to take in carbohydrate, mostly in the form of liquids from a high-glycemic-index source. The best choice is your favorite sports drink. You could also use gels chased immediately by lots of water. The longer the workout, the more important carbohydrate is. For an hour or less of training, water is all you need, assuming you put something in the tank during stage 1. As the workout gets longer, the amount of carbohydrate you take in per hour also increases. This could be as few as 100 calories or as many as 400 calories per hour depending not »

Continued

only on workout length but also on body size, workout intensity, and your experience.

STAGE 3 Immediately after the workout

This and the next stage are the key times in the day for taking in carbohydrate. When athletes say that eating in stages doesn't work for them, it's nearly always because they don't take in enough carbohydrate in stages 3 and 4.

Your purpose now is to replace the carbohydrate you used up during the workout. In the first 30 minutes or so after a high-dose workout, your body is several hundred times more sensitive to carbohydrate than at any other time of the day. The longer you wait to refuel, the less likely you are to completely refill the tank. Take in 3 to 4 calories per pound of body weight, mostly from carbohydrate, during this stage.

You can buy a commercial product for this, although they are expensive. Or you can make your own by blending about 16 ounces of fruit juice with a banana; 3 to 5 tablespoons of glucose, such as Carbo-Pro (available at sportquestdirect.com), depending on body size; and 30 to 40 grams of protein powder, especially from egg or whey sources. Drinking this in the 30-minute postworkout window is critical for recovery. It should be your highest priority after a hard workout. If the workout was low dose, though, omit this stage.

STAGE 4 As long as the workout lasted

For the next several minutes, or as long as the preceding workout lasted, continue to focus your diet on carbohydrate, especially from moderate- to high-glycemic-index sources, along with some protein. You may be ready to eat a meal during stage 4 if the workout was long. Now is also the time to eat starches such as pasta, bread, bagels, cereal, rice, corn, » and other foods rich in fast-absorbing glucose to maintain the recovery process. Perhaps the perfect foods to eat at this time are potatoes, sweet potatoes, yams, and bananas. And a great snack food for stage 4 is raisins. Eat until satisfied, being careful not to overeat, which is possible when enjoying sweet-tasting carbs.

STAGE 5 **Until the next workout**

Now you're at work, spending time with the family, maintaining your landscaping or whatever it is you do when not training or racing on a given day of the week. Although this part of your day may look ordinary to the rest of the world, it really isn't. You're still focused on nutrition for long-term recovery.

This is the time when many athletes get sloppy with their diets. The most common mistake is continuing to eat a diet that is low in nutrient value and high in starch and sugar, as was common in stages 3 and 4. Such foods are relatively poor in vitamins and minerals. The most nutrient-dense foods are vegetables, fruits, and lean protein from animal sources, especially seafood. Snack on nuts, seeds, and berries. All of these foods are rich in vitamins, minerals, and other trace elements necessary for health, growth, and recovery.

• • •

Avoid foods that come in packages, including those with labels that say "healthy." They aren't. If your great-great-grandmother couldn't have eaten it, then it is best avoided. That includes foods invented by sports nutrition scientists. Just eat real food in stage 5.

If you are doing two or three workouts in a day, you may not get to stage 5 until late in the day. Also, stage 4 may replace stage 1 with closely spaced workouts. That's not a problem.

sidebar "Eating for Recovery on a High-Carb Diet" provides a quick summary of the common recovery methods to follow relative to exercise when eating a high-carb diet.

When fat is the primary macronutrient in the daily diet, however, ketones, not glucose, are the primary energy source. Ketones are produced by the liver from fat. For the athlete on a high-fat/low-carbohydrate diet, there is little in the way of glucose available; ketone production increases, and the athlete is said to be in a state of "ketosis" (not to be confused with "ketoacidosis," which is a serious medical condition sometimes experienced by type 1 diabetics). The skeletal muscles along with the heart, brain, and other vital organs function normally on ketones once the body adapts, which can take a few weeks.

Since even the skinniest athlete has plenty of stored body fat, the source of energy is unlikely to run out during endurance events lasting even several hours. So in-race refueling is not an issue, as it is when eating a high-carb diet. For example, many ultramarathon runners follow a high-fat diet and take in little or no fuel during events of 50 kilometers (31 miles) or more.

Recovery is also simple on a high-fat diet. Normal meals and snacks, made up primarily of fat, are eaten after workouts with no need to consume "extra" fat. There's also no need for "loading" before a long race.

You can't mix the two diets—it's either a high-carb or a high-fat diet if you are to perform well. The body preferentially depends on either fat or sugar for fueling your aerobic exercise based on which it receives the most of on a daily basis. Eat a lot of carbohydrate, and the body burns a lot of sugar. Eat mostly fat, and the body is fueled mostly with fat. You also must follow the standard rules for recovery on your chosen diet. Eating a high-fat diet but recovering with lots of sugar is counterproductive, and recovering with fat on a high-carb diet won't cut it, either.

In Chapter 8 we'll get into the types of foods that make up these chronic diets and the relative benefits of both. First, however, let's look into the role of protein in recovery and its implications for the senior athlete.

Protein and Recovery

While the number of studies on the topics of food, recovery, and aging is small, all of those studies seem to indicate that older athletes need more protein, especially during recovery, than younger athletes do.[31] There is evidence to suggest that we don't synthesize—meaning process in order to rebuild tissues—protein as well as we get older, especially for the restructuring of the slow-twitch endurance muscles.[32] The older athlete, therefore, needs more protein to ensure that there is enough to help with the rebuilding that takes place during sleep. It also appears that on the days of strength training and intervals, eating some protein about 30 minutes before going to bed helps to stimulate muscle building, at least in young athletes.[33] This dovetails very nicely with what you read earlier regarding the University of North Dakota study on macronutrient choices late in the day to improve sleep.[34] But bear in mind that a large late-evening snack may conflict with falling asleep, as we saw earlier.[35]

Since simply eating more total calories in order to take in additional protein isn't a good way to increase this food type, it implies that there is a reduced need for either carbohydrate or fat with aging. We'll return to that topic in Chapter 8.

Protein has other benefits for the aging athlete when it comes to recovery. A 2014 review of the scientific literature related to protein intake and exercise by Stuart Phillips of McMaster University in Canada showed that when and how much protein you take in after a workout, especially a strength-building session such as lifting weights, has a lot to do with how beneficial the workout is for the muscles.[36] To build or even just to maintain muscle mass, the rate of muscle protein synthesis must be greater than the rate of muscle protein breakdown as it happens during and after a strength workout. Fortunately, strength training stimulates muscle protein synthesis. But without adequate dietary protein to support this rebuilding process, the body is forced to "cannibalize" itself by taking protein from lightly used muscles to rebuild the highly stressed muscles. This suggests the need to take in protein after workouts to meet the body's needs.

And it just so happens that eating protein also increases the rate of muscle rebuilding, especially if it's eaten *immediately* after exercise. The benefit decreases the longer you wait. So I recommend that after a strength workout or any session that is highly stressful to the muscles, such as aerobic-capacity or lactate-threshold intervals, you eat some protein within 30 minutes of finishing. How much?

In reviewing the research on how much protein should be eaten, Dr. Phillips found that older athletes need a lot. While a young athlete benefits from eating 20 to 25 grams (about 80 to 100 calories) of protein after a workout, older athletes may need 40 grams (about 160 calories) to achieve the same level of muscle protein synthesis.[37] Consuming 160 calories from protein is equivalent to eating about six boiled eggs (with 6.29 g of protein per egg) after a workout. That's a lot of eggs. It may be less difficult to get your protein by also including protein powder in your postworkout recovery drink. In that case I'd recommend using egg- or whey-based protein powder.

There are several amino acids in foods that together make up what we call protein. The individual amino acid that has been shown to be the most beneficial for muscle rebuilding during recovery is leucine,[38] which has many good sources including whole eggs, egg whites, egg protein powder, and whey protein. Egg protein powder, however, can be quite expensive. Besides eggs, other common foods relatively high in leucine are most all dairy products, all animal products, dried figs, pasta, spinach, buttermilk, most nuts, most seeds, coconut milk and cream, avocado, most beans, corn, peas, spirulina, and succotash. These are good food choices for your postworkout recovery snack and the next meal after a hard workout to boost protein and leucine intake and muscle rebuilding.

Other Recovery Aids

There are many other methods typically used by athletes to enhance recovery that we'll explore next. Some of these may be more effective for you than others, as there is a fair amount of individuality when it comes to recovery aids. Note, however, that none of these approach the level of recovery benefits of sleep and nutrition. Those must always be your primary focus when recovering between high-dose workouts or during periodic Rest and Recovery breaks.

The recovery methods and devices discussed here are commonly used and mostly research-supported. For some, though, a few studies found no recovery benefit at all. When that happens, it tells us something—the benefits are so small that they may not always be measurable or even occurring.

What we'll consider here is not an all-inclusive list but only the most common. There may be other methods that work for you just as well or perhaps even better. If that's the case, by all means continue to use them regardless of what the research may or may not say. For example, there's little research on elevating your legs after a workout to speed recovery, yet it is quite commonly and successfully used. In the same way, light exercise while using flotation devices in a swimming pool is effectively used by many. Listening to music after exercise has even been shown to promote recovery, at least in youngsters.[39] It isn't taken too seriously by those who study recovery, but do what works best for you.

Something else to note is that most of the following recovery modes were studied using young males—mainly college students—and in some cases nonathletes. So the methods I'm going to explain here may be less applicable or effective for us older athletes. Also, a lot of the supportive research was based on study designs in which very-short-term recovery was the focus. For example, the subjects did two hard workouts on the same day with different types of recovery between them to see which resulted in the best performance in the second exercise session. Two-a-day workouts may never be a concern for you. The bottom line is that it's a good idea to be a bit skeptical when it comes to things that have been shown to marginally improve recovery. Basically, science knows less about nonsleep and non-nutrition recovery than appears to be the case if you read the advertisements for such products.[40] Your experience counts for a lot when it comes to recovery techniques.

Active Recovery

Active recovery is probably the most common method employed by all athletes. It involves light exercise using low intensity and short duration after a high-dose workout. An example would be a cyclist going for an easy bike ride on his or her recovery day following an interval session the day before. Or perhaps a runner doing light running-simulation exercise in the deep end of a pool while wearing a flotation device. Active recovery probably works best for athletes with a high level of aerobic fitness.[41] If marginally trained athletes use active recovery, the workout dosage needs to be much lower than that for the highly trained.[42]

Passive Recovery

If active recovery is more effective for the highly trained athlete, then it stands to reason that passive recovery—complete rest, as in a day off without a workout—is better for those who are less well trained. Regardless of your fitness level, inactivity—total rest—is great for recovery.[43] It's also the best option for those new to endurance sport or making a comeback after a long layoff. While there appears to be no supporting research, it's likely that the older you are, the more passive recovery you need.

Compression Garments

In the early 2000s, compression garments, especially stockings, were borrowed from medicine by athletes as a new recovery device. Since then, their use has continued to grow. They've also been used by athletes during races and workouts to improve performance, although this use has not been well supported by the research.[44] Of course, if you sense that wearing a compression garment improves your performance, by all means continue to use it. There is no apparent downside. There are a few studies showing that if compression garments are worn during recovery (and in some cases also during the preceding workout), muscle soreness is decreased[45] and subsequent exercise performance is improved.[46] This postworkout recovery method is relatively inexpensive and worth a try.

Pneumatic Compression Devices

You may have seen a pneumatic compression device in a physical therapy clinic, and you may even know an athlete who owns one. It comprises sleeves that slip over the legs (or, less commonly, the arms) and are then hooked up to a small pneumatic pump. The pump inflates chambers in the sleeves, starting at the farthest end, followed by each subsequent chamber going up the leg (or arm). The sleeves then deflate and start all over again. Settings control how long one cycle takes and how much pressure is produced. The purpose is to speed up the removal of the metabolic waste products of exercise such as lactate, ammonia, and pyruvate. Common brand names as of this writing are NormaTec, Recovery Boot, and Flowtron. The use of these devices for many medical conditions such as deep-vein thrombosis[47] is well supported, but there is limited research on their use by athletes. What research does exist seems to support their benefits in terms of both recovery[48] and subsequent performance after an exhaustive workout.[49] As you might expect, such devices are considerably more expensive than the others described here.

Cold Water and Contrasting Water Therapy

After a high-intensity workout, you can immerse the overworked muscles in cold water or alternate between hot and cold water for a few minutes to speed recovery.[50] Both of these techniques have been shown to be more effective than either passive recovery or hot-water immersion. For cold immersion, the temperature should be 50° to 60°F (10° to 15° C) and for hot about 100° to 104°F (38° to 40°C).[51] The same research indicates that only about 6 to 15 minutes of total immersion time for either the cold or contrasting-temperature method is all that's needed. More time doesn't appear to make recovery any better.

I recall back in the 1970s being introduced to the idea of putting an icepack on muscles after a hard workout to speed recovery. Now it appears that this may actually delay recovery.[52] The times, they are a-changing.

Muscle Manipulation

This category includes both massage and foam rollers, which have become very popular in the past several years. There isn't much research on foam

Plucking Myths: Aging Cyclists and Improved Performance

JOHN HOWARD

Many people think masters athletes recover more slowly than their younger counterparts. I am not one of them. Current evidence may support me.

A January 12, 2014, *Wall Street Journal* article by Robbie Shell is an illustration in point. It includes an interview between Shell and 70-year-old cyclist Michael Patterson, a retired JP Morgan Chase executive, and Brent Rudy, director of the Center for Work Physiology and Exercise Metabolism at the University of Montana. The article recalls the efforts of Patterson's four-man team, all aged 70 and older, during the 2012 Race Across America (RAAM). The team covered the distance in six and a half days, setting a new 60-and-above age record. An interesting comparison was made in the interview using a previous overall record time, set in 2008, that was just *two and a half hours* faster than Patterson's team's time. The 2008 team, using a training program similar to that followed by the 70-year-olds, consumed only slightly more calories for their effort. The critical difference was age. The 2008 team's average age was only 37! Rudy makes a point for reconsidering some of the inherent limitations that we may place upon ourselves when considering the mystique of aging: "We clearly need to rethink our ideas about what older people are capable of doing, yet we discount those capabilities all the time. As people get older, they can still do amazing things."

I am one of the original founders of RAAM and a former participant. I believe that while endurance training and racing seems to be a viable competitive arena for more active older athletes, there is no denial of our limitations. Among the limits is maximum output; since I have been competing, I have taken the time to have my vital capacities measured every decade of my life since my 20s. The raw scores are, in and of themselves, not encouraging. I have lost more than 23 percent of »

Continued

my VO$_2$max score, the measure of human horsepower. My power-per-kilogram numbers have also suffered. Yet, at 66, I still have a category I racing license and can still hold my own against the younger dudes during both training rides and races. How is this possible? As a coach, I use a formula for finding a cyclist's inherent weaknesses. Irrespective of age, each of us needs to find these weaknesses and address them.

Here is what I've come to understand about masters cyclists. It is important to know your power numbers—monitoring power plays a role in the total performance equation, but it is one of a number of important data points. Far more important is finding your personal idiosyncrasies that affect range of motion (ROM) and strength. Body work, using therapies such as dynamic motion or active release, can pinpoint soft-tissue impingements that affect the ability to produce power. Systematic balancing of power from both sides of the body is critical, as is linear force vectoring. Once ROM has improved, strength training needs to support the precise motor action of pedaling. A customized program that addresses each individual's unique flexibility and strength issues is an absolute must for improvement. When you lose nearly a quarter of your vital capacity, you need to be spot-on with your training regimen and　»

rollers when it comes to recovery from exercise. But what is available indicates that muscle soreness is reduced and range of motion increased when a roller is used immediately after a hard workout.[53] To use a foam roller, lie or sit with the belly of the muscle needing recovery on the roller and then roll back and forth on it so that the entire length of the muscle is manipulated by the pressure.

Massage has been the subject of a great many studies, with varying results in terms of recovery. That may be because there is a wide array

your bike position. By using this approach, many athletes have found that their power numbers and overall performance have improved even as they age.

I am but one example. As I have aged, I have actually improved my "hinge," as I call it, thus making my 6-foot, 2-inch body more aero than those of most cyclists standing 5 to 6 inches less. My setup allows me a flattened upper torso stretched out over the bike, which not only brings the core into play but also improves my sustainable cruise speed by up to 2 mph under ideal conditions. The core activation saves the big muscles from drawing down too much power too quickly by creating added stability, thus reducing heart rate.

When we talk about diminished recovery for masters athletes, let's tell the truth about what is actually happening. One bodily function may regress, but if we train correctly with an individual plan, other workable functions rise to take up the slack. While I've lost VO_2 capacity, I have increased flexibility and strength, replaced missing nutritional essentials, and generally made myself a better-rounded athlete.

I welcome your input. For more observations, please see my book *Mastering Cycling.*

of methods called "massage," and there may be great variability in the masseurs' techniques and abilities. It's also hard to control the placebo benefits for study subjects when it comes to *not* getting a massage. Consequently, only a few recent studies have shown subsequent reduced muscle soreness and performance improvement from deep massage after stressful exercise.[54] But some scientists who have reviewed all of the available research studies have also concluded that there are no physical benefits.[55] Of course, the benefits may well be psychological, which, I suppose, is nearly as good as physical when it comes to feeling recovered. Massage can certainly be relaxing.

Nutrition and Body Composition

As we have seen in this chapter, nutrition is a key component in our recovery and rebuilding from exercise. Arguably, proper nutrition is more critical to the senior athlete's performance than it is for younger athletes. It also appears that as we get older we need more protein in our diets to help maintain or even build muscle. Without adequate protein, we are more likely to experience a loss of muscle and therefore strength and power. This contributes to the slowing that aging athletes experience. It's not the only reason we get slower, but it's one of them.

Beyond recovery, though, we also need to think about how what we eat influences our body composition. As you've undoubtedly discovered, age brings with it its own thoughts on what your body should look like and how it should be shaped. Fighting the accumulation of tissue and keeping body fat at bay can become a full-time job once we've passed 60. In fact, the whole matter of nutrition and aging demands a more in-depth examination. That will be a topic in the next chapter as we return to the last of the big three causes for our reduced performance with aging: increasing body fat.

BODY FAT

You aren't old until age becomes your excuse.

—JOE FRIEL

Things change as we age. When I was 50, I had absolutely no problem maintaining a very low, steady, and healthy level of body fat. According to the fit of my clothes and my waist circumference, there had been no change since I was in college (I even still had some of my college clothes, to my wife's chagrin), and I was actually somewhat leaner at age 50 than I had been at 20. In fact, it wasn't until my mid-60s that I began to see a change in my body makeup. Around then I started getting a bit of a belly every winter. Not huge, mind you, but certainly unusual for me. Despite my training load staying similar to what it had been just a few years before, my body had begun to change, and I, in turn, needed to change something to stay ahead of my growing belly. There were several options available, and in studying and experimenting with them, I became much smarter about how my aging body works.

If you're also experiencing this change in body fat, you have the same options. We've covered some of them already: changing your workouts to focus more on intensity, doing more strength work, changing your periodization by, perhaps, going to a nine-day "week" (as described in Chapter 6), or simply doing a better job of recovering between challenging workouts and in Rest and Recovery breaks. Some of these routines may work better for you than others, as I learned. But there are additional ways to maintain your leanness or possibly even reverse the physical consequences of increasing fat with aging, and that's where we want to go in this chapter.

Measuring Body Fat

What we're discussing here is not body weight but rather *body composition.* It's common for aging people, especially men, to lose weight as they add excess fat to their bodies.[1] That's because they are losing muscle while adding fat. Since muscle is more dense than fat, you can slowly add a lot of fat while losing some muscle, and it will appear, at least on your bathroom scale, that everything is OK. Weight is a somewhat better indicator of increasing body fat for women—their muscle mass does not decline much because their starting point was typically much lower than a man's.[2]

Body composition is about the relative percentages of lean and fat mass in your body, and as we'll see later, there are several different ways to measure it. The lean part includes muscles, tendons, ligaments, bones, organs, water—everything that isn't fat. Fat is also known as adipose tissue and is either of the white or brown variety. Brown fat in adults is found in the upper back, along the neck, in the shoulder, and along the spine.[3] It's there to protect you from the cold. The contribution of brown fat to the metabolic rate—calorie burning—is second only to that of the muscles. Just as with muscle, the brown fat content of the body decreases with age. That's why we typically feel colder as we get older. The loss of brown fat is not really a problem unless you spend a lot of time in a cold environment. It's the white fat we need to address when it comes to body composition.

White fat stores energy, which of course is necessary for a healthy life. It's just that as we get older, the trend is to sock away increasing amounts of energy. Science is not yet sure why this occurs with aging; for now, the most we can say is that it just happens. Still, as an athlete, you probably have nowhere near the energy-storage capacity—the flab, that is—of your sedentary neighbor. For "normal" inactive men, white body fat may make up about 20 percent of their weight; for sedentary women, the figure is roughly 25 percent. And that, mind you, is only if they are overweight and not obese, at which point the numbers become staggering (and unfortunately all too common these days). There isn't much research on this topic, but the little there is suggests that sedentary men in their late 60s carry about nine more pounds of fat than do similarly aged athletes.[4] An even greater difference was found for older female athletes versus older nonathletic women—about 17 pounds.[5] This is one reason why those who study healthy aging are so interested in the lifestyles of athletes.

One of the major concerns for most athletes is how much white fat they are hauling around the course on race day. Among endurance athletes, perhaps only open-water swimmers benefit from excess storage of white fat, since it insulates their bodies from the cold and supplies some buoyancy. For other endurance sports, though, excess fat is generally a performance inhibitor. Too much of it means you are slower, especially when working against gravity. One pound of excess weight costs roughly 2 watts on a bike hill climb and 2 seconds per mile while running. Runners are especially sensitive to the constraints of excess blubber due to the vertical oscillation—bouncing—that is normal in running. Raising the center of the runner's body by a few centimeters with every stride takes more energy and effort if there is excess weight.

Athletes commonly want to know how much extra fat they have. "Extra" in this context means above and beyond what is necessary for health. For youthful, elite endurance athletes, a common body-fat percentage is typically about 6 percent of total body weight for men and 12 percent for women. These percentages are very close to the lowest limits considered by experts to be healthy.[6] They may vary by a couple of percentage points up or down, depending on the sport, time of the season, and the individual. The fastest senior athletes carry somewhat more fat, perhaps 5 to 8 percent more than the lightest elite athletes. Yet all of these figures are still considered lean by society's standards.

While weight is critical to success, it can be a tricky metric. Your bathroom scale may not be a very good indicator of what's actually going on with your body since as we age, muscle is generally lost while fat is gained. The net result may show no change on the scale, or it may even show a loss of weight. The number may look good, but it could be masking what's really happening over time. But you can make your scale a better tool for determining changes in fat by getting a body-composition measurement, as described below. This measurement will reveal your body-fat percentage. Once you have that number, you can multiply it by total body weight to find the weight of your fat. Subtract that from total body weight, and you know the lean weight of your body.

As mentioned earlier, your lean weight includes lots of stuff besides muscle. However, muscle is the most likely to change significantly over time, so you can be relatively sure that increases or decreases in leanness are caused by changes in muscle. Periodic measurements of body composition, perhaps a couple of times a year, allow you to determine how your muscle-building strength workouts and your fat-control methods (which we'll discuss soon) are going. In between measurements, you can assume that body composition remains stable. That means changes in body weight on your bathroom scale can be fairly reliably converted to changes in fat and muscle. After weighing at a standard time every day, such as on waking in the morning, you can use a calculator to determine fat stores.

There are several ways to measure body composition. Some are more accurate than others. They also vary in availability, cost, and ease of implementation. The most common method uses calipers to measure pinched fat deposits at certain points on the body. These measurements are then poured into a formula that determines fat mass. A technician does all of this for you. Because this is the cheapest and probably the easiest measurement to obtain, I recommend going this route. Caliper measurements are typically performed at health clubs and medical clinics, or your coach may offer one. The key to reliable numbers is to have the same person do the measurements each time. That will cancel out most of the error that can occur with this method.

More accurate but more expensive (and less widely available) measurement methods are bioelectrical impedance, which passes an electrical flow through the body; underwater weighing, which takes advantage of the fact that fat floats; air displacement (which is similar to underwater weighing); and Dual Energy X-ray Absorptiometry (DEXA or, more commonly these days, DXA), considered to be the gold standard for accuracy.

In addition to these body composition measurement methods, other easy measures of fatness that roughly estimate changes in body fat can be used if you'd prefer not to feel like a lab rat with someone pinching and measuring your fat stores. All you need do is measure your waist periodically, since that is where older men and women store the most fat.[7] The fit of your pants and belts around the waist are also indicators of the direction your fatness is going. If your waist size is increasing, you are more than likely gaining fat regardless of what your scale may report. Of course, what we'd like to see is the opposite—a gradual reduction in waist girth over time. If that happens and you are still gaining weight or it's staying the same, then you are adding muscle. Determining body composition by monitoring weight does not deliver results that are even close to the accuracy you'd get from a pinch-and-caliper measurement, but it is certainly available and cheap.

Unfortunately, it's common with age to experience an increase in body fat and a decrease in muscle. The possible contributors to the increase in body fat are diet; training; menopause; medications; and, of course, our old friend hormones. We'll examine each of these to get a sense of what you can do, or avoid doing, to better manage your body composition. Let's start with hormones since they have such a great impact on how the others benefit or detract from your body composition.

Hormones

You may recall that in Chapter 3 I told you about an enzyme called lipoprotein lipase (LPL) that plays a critical role in causing your body to store fat. Wherever LPL is found in abundance, your body will store fat if given the chance. For men, that location throughout life is primarily in the belly. For women, it shifts around a bit. When a woman is young, much of her LPL is found on the hips and butt, but after menopause it shifts to the belly.

When you were younger, the fat-storing activity of LPL was limited by your testosterone levels (which are, of course, much greater in men than in women). But as you've gotten older, as we've discussed, your testosterone production has decreased.[8] So with advancing age the capability of your LPL to stockpile fat has increased. The result is that you are likely storing more fat as the years go by.[9] Unfortunately, the reason that it may be evolutionarily necessary for older people to store larger amounts of fat than younger people is as yet unknown.

In addition to testosterone, other hormones play a role in the activity of LPL. While testosterone decreases LPL's fat-storing activity, insulin increases it. Insulin is a hormone produced by the pancreas that, among other things, causes muscle and fat cells to absorb glucose, a sugar, from the blood. After a carbohydrate-rich meal, especially one that includes high-glycemic-load foods that cause a rapid increase in blood sugar (I'll explain this further in the following section), insulin is released. While insulin is often considered a "bad boy" for its effects on fatness, it plays a critical role in health. If it weren't for insulin, the blood-sugar increase after eating would result in health problems, which is the situation faced daily by type 1 diabetics. On the other hand, too much insulin production (which can result, in part, from a high consumption of sugary foods) causes the body, mostly the muscle cells, to lose sensitivity to the hormone. When that happens, the pancreas works overtime to produce insulin in an attempt to remove sugar from the blood. At some point it becomes unsuccessful, as there is just too much sugar to be stored. Production of insulin reaches its upper limit. The upshot is that the body loses its sensitivity to insulin, resulting in what's known as "insulin resistance" and the early stages of type 2 diabetes. Some people are much more genetically prone to this than others. There are many health consequences of this condition, frequently resulting in a shortened life span. And with advancing age, type 2 diabetics are at increased risk of dementia such as Alzheimer's disease.[10] Fortunately, regular exercise increases the body's sensitivity to insulin, reducing the potential for overproduction and its associated problems.[11]

Given your long-standing level of exercise, you are probably not at risk of type 2 diabetes.[12] But while regular exercise over many years may reduce the risk of type 2 diabetes, it does not stop the activity of LPL and the potential accumulation of fat.[13] Nor does it inhibit the activities of the hormones that cause hunger and satiety—leptin and ghrelin. Both of these hormones also play a role in insulin production and therefore fat accumulation with aging.

"Leptin" and "ghrelin" might sound like terms from a television sci-fi show; it may help to know that "leptin" comes from the Greek term *leptos*, for "thin," while ghrelin is an acronym derived from its description as a *g*rowth *h*ormone *rel*ease-*in*ducing peptide. Leptin is the "satiety hormone." When it is produced, your hunger for food decreases. You feel satisfied. Ghrelin is the "hunger hormone." When its production increases, you feel the need to eat. When your stomach is empty, or nearly so, ghrelin is released; when it is full and stretched, ghrelin production stops, and leptin steps in.[14]

The interplay of these hormones throughout the day helps to regulate energy balance; ideally, your energy intake equals your energy output and storage. For some unknown reason, women produce more ghrelin than men do, regardless of their age,[15] but also experience an increase in leptin levels with advancing age.[16] Fortunately, aerobic exercise has been shown to reduce the activity of both ghrelin and leptin, thus reducing the hunger-satiety swings.[17]

Is there anything else you can do about this interplay of insulin, leptin, and ghrelin? Science is still discovering the answers to that question. One of the known conditions that plays a role in managing these hormones takes us back to a recovery topic in Chapter 7: sleep.[18] (There are others, such as becoming obese—something you'd probably rather not do, but which, paradoxically, has been found to decrease the production of insulin.[19]) Recall from the previous chapter that testosterone is released during sleep, especially in the latter portion of a full night's snooze. And since

TIM
NOAKES,
MD

Insulin Resistance

Insulin resistance (IR), or carbohydrate intolerance (CI), is, in my opinion, a hereditary trait or predisposition that is present to varying degrees in a large proportion of modern humans. Its widespread distribution in peoples on all continents suggests that it must have been of significant evolutionary survival value. IR is a condition in which the body has an impaired capacity to safely metabolize and store ingested carbohydrate.

Humans are not the only mammals to exhibit IR. Any carnivorous species is likely to be IR, and the cat family appears to be especially affected. Since IR is a necessary factor leading to type 2 diabetes mellitus (T2DM), it is not surprising that, like humans, domesticated cats and captive African lions are also experiencing an epidemic increase in T2DM (and obesity)—and for the same reasons.

Visible external evidence of IR becomes increasingly apparent with age, generally beginning to show as increased difficulty in controlling body mass in middle age, leading to obesity; high blood pressure; and the metabolic syndrome, including T2DM. Factors that worsen IR with age probably include diets high in sugar, high-fructose corn syrup, and other carbohydrates, aggravated perhaps by low levels of habitual physical activity.

The common abnormality in IR is resistance of the liver to the action of insulin. Insulin regulates the rate at which the liver produces glucose from fat and protein or stores blood glucose derived from the digestion of ingested carbohydrate. But in IR the liver does not properly "recognize" insulin. As a result, the livers of persons with IR overproduce glucose 24 hours a day; this is the immediate cause of the raised blood glucose concentrations in T2DM.

The liver and muscles of persons with IR also have a reduced capacity to store glucose. As a consequence, when a person with IR »

Continued

ingests a high-carbohydrate meal, the blood glucose concentration rises excessively, requiring the oversecretion of insulin to remove the added glucose from the bloodstream. This is necessary because glucose in high concentration is toxic to all the cells of the body. But if the glucose load from the ingested carbohydrate cannot be stored in the liver or muscles, it will be converted to fat (triglyceride) in the liver and transported as triglyceride in the bloodstream to the fat cells. In this way, the toxic substance, glucose, is converted and stored as a somewhat less toxic substance, fat. But when too much fat is stored, it too can begin to have detrimental effects.

Two other abnormalities present in those with IR when they ingest high-carbohydrate diets are low blood HDL cholesterol concentrations and increased numbers of small, dense LDL cholesterol particles in the bloodstream. There is abundant evidence clearly showing that these biological markers of IR (and of a habitual high-carbohydrate diet)—elevated blood glucose; insulin and triglyceride concentrations; low HDL cholesterol concentrations; and increased numbers of small, dense LDL-cholesterol particles—are also the best predictors of heart attack risk and perhaps of other diseases such as cancer and dementia.

What does all this mean?

First, that it is excess carbohydrate, not fat, in the diet that is causing the epidemic of chronic diseases, including obesity and T2DM, that first began in 1980, three years after the new U.S. dietary guidelines promoting a low-fat, high-carbohydrate diet were first promulgated.

Second, that the amount of carbohydrate each of us can safely metabolize is determined by our individual degree of IR. In my opinion, the range of safe daily carbohydrate intake goes from 25 to 200 grams per day, depending on each individual's degree of IR. To optimize their health, those with T2DM and who are the most IR must restrict their carbohydrate intakes to about 25 g/day, whereas those who are without »

IR can safely ingest 200 g/day. But in my opinion, there is never any need to ingest more carbohydrate, even if one is exercising for many hours a day. Humans evolved as fat-burning athletes without any essential requirement for even a single gram of ingested carbohydrate to keep us active and healthy. In my opinion, we are the most healthy when we return to that state.

To conclude: For 33 years I followed and advocated through my book, *Lore of Running*, the current dogma that to be active and healthy, one must eat a diet low in fat and high in carbohydrate. I now believe that this advice was quite wrong. I apologize. It was an honest error.

But if, like me, you have IR, I hope you will take my apology to heart and, for the sake of your future health, consider limiting the amount of carbohydrate that you include in your diet. You may be amazed by the transformation in your health that this simple dietary change can produce.

testosterone limits the activity of the fat-storing enzyme LPL, a bit more sleep every day may help to keep your waist trim and the caliper pinches small. Sleep also plays a role in regulating the levels of ghrelin and leptin. So if you're not getting enough sleep, you may feel like eating more, especially sugary junk food.[20] Managing body fat may be as simple as sleeping a little longer.

We've previously examined testosterone production relative to your training. You learned that vigorous, high-intensity workouts have been shown to result in more androgenic hormone production,[21] such as LPL-limiting testosterone. This is another instance of how lifting heavy weights and doing aerobic-capacity intervals may provide a performance benefit by not only improving the muscular and aerobic systems but also reducing the storage of fat.

I've mentioned it several times, so now is a good time to take a look at the elephant in the room—the relationship between what you eat and how much body fat you have.

Diet

There is no perfect diet that works for all athletes. I wish I could tell you there is, but the fact is, personalized nutrition is the key. When it comes to body composition, health, recovery, and athletic performance, you need to eat a diet that's right for you. So how do you choose among the many possible common diets and food selections? The starting point is to determine how the diet you currently eat is working. You can do that by considering how your body is functioning in several areas. Here are some pertinent questions to ask:

- Am I becoming fatter, as indicated by technician-measured changes in total body composition (such as calipers or DEXA) or by my measured increases in belly fat?
- Do I have frequent illnesses, especially upper-respiratory problems such as head colds and sore throats?
- Is my recovery from high-dose workouts unusually slow compared with how quickly I recovered from similar workouts just a couple of years ago?
- Compared with a few years ago, are my training and race performances declining at a faster rate, as marked by fatigue, poor endurance, and declining results?
- Have I experienced a measurable loss of muscular strength over the past year or so?

- Have I been told by my doctor that I am obese, am prediabetic, have high blood pressure, or am at high risk for heart disease?

If you don't answer yes to any of these questions, your current diet is probably correct for you. Keep it up. But bear in mind that things can change with advancing age, and frequently do. For example, we know that as you age, your LPL becomes more sensitive to insulin because there is a reduction in the testosterone available to keep it from storing fat. In other words, you more easily convert high-glycemic-load foods to fat. That's the second time I've mentioned high glycemic load. So what does that mean? This is a topic that may have a bearing on your fat storage.

Glycemic Load

Glycemic load (GL) is a way of gauging how fast and how much the carbohydrate in the food you eat raises your blood-sugar levels. It's a better indicator than a gauge called glycemic index, which measures only how quickly blood sugar rises after eating carbohydrate. The more sugar there is in the food *and* the more rapidly sugar enters the bloodstream, the higher the GL of that food. This is important because, as you read earlier, when your body senses a rapid rise in blood sugar, it takes action. Your pancreas produces insulin to sock the sugar away in muscles that are low in glycogen (one of the body's forms of stored sugar), as they might be after a recent workout. Your body may also convert the sugar to fat and store it in fat tissues, including the ones on your belly. As we get older, our muscles become somewhat less sensitive to insulin, but our fat cells do not. So the sugar is more likely to wind up on your belly. That contributes to gaining fat with age.

The glycemic load of a given food is measured on a scale of 0 to 50; foods with a number greater than 20 are considered "high," 11 to 19 are rated "medium," and 10 or less are called "low." The higher the GL of your food choices, the greater your risk of increasing body fat, among other negative health implications. Note that the GL rating of the food alone is not necessarily the cause of an increase in body fat. At least one study using young men as subjects did not find that to be the case.[22] Instead, the correlation may be that high-GL food causes a craving that can easily result in overeating such foods.[23] Regardless of the mechanism, low-GL diets have been shown to result in a loss of total body fat and weight.[24] Table 8.1 lists the GL of common foods.[25]

Note that Table 8.1 does not rate foods with regard to how healthy they are. Just because ice cream has a low GL of 6 doesn't mean that it's healthier to eat lots of it while avoiding grapes, which have a moderate GL of 11. You're more likely to pig out on ice cream than on grapes. Table 8.1 is meant only as a guide for determining the sugar spike that the food creates when you eat a serving of it. It also doesn't tell us anything about what the other health implications of the food may be. For example, the vitamin and mineral contents of foods are not reflected in this table. That said, if you answered yes to any of the questions in the earlier list, you may want to consider eating fewer moderate- and high-GL foods and make more low-GL choices.

Changing Your Diet

I've made several comments about the possible need to change your diet as you get older since physiology shifts in the body over time. Your dietary needs had little relationship to physical performance when you were a teenager. My, how things have changed now. A 50-year-old has a greatly different set of needs when it comes to eating. You should also realize that

TABLE 8.1. The Glycemic Load of 68 Common Foods by Category

FOOD	GLYCEMIC LOAD PER SERVING	FOOD	GLYCEMIC LOAD PER SERVING
Bakery Product and Bread		**Cookies and Crackers**	
Bagel, white, frozen	25	Graham crackers	14
Baguette, white, plain	15	Rice cakes	17
Bread, whole wheat	9	Soda crackers	12
Corn tortilla	12	Vanilla wafers	14
Hamburger bun	9	**Dairy**	
Vanilla cake	24	Ice cream	6
Beverages		Milk, full fat	5
Apple juice, unsweetened	30	Milk, skim	4
Coca Cola	16	Reduced-fat yogurt with fruit	11
Gatorade	12		
Orange juice, unsweetened	12	**Fruits**	
Tomato juice, canned	4	Apple	6
Breakfast Cereals		Banana	16
Cornflakes	23	Grapefruit	3
Coco Pops	20	Grapes	11
Cream of Wheat	17	Orange	4
Grapenuts	16	Peach	5
Instant oatmeal	30	Pear	4
Muesli	16	Raisins	28
Puffed wheat	17	Watermelon	4
Raisin Bran	12	**Beans and Nuts**	
Special K	14	Baked beans	6
Grains		Black beans	7
Brown rice	16	Cashews, salted	3
Corn on the cob	20	Kidney beans	7
Couscous	9	Lentils	5
Quinoa	13	Navy beans	9
White rice	43	Peanuts	0
		Soy beans	1

Continued

Continued

FOOD	GLYCEMIC LOAD PER SERVING	FOOD	GLYCEMIC LOAD PER SERVING
Pasta and Noodles		**Vegetables**	
Fettucini	15	Carrots	2
Macaroni and cheese	32	Baked russet potato	33
Spaghetti, white, boiled 20 min.	26	Boiled white potato	21
Spaghetti, whole meal	17	Instant mashed potato	17
Snack Foods		Sweet potato	22
		Yam	20
Corn chips	11	**Miscellaneous**	
Potato chips	12	Chicken nuggets, frozen	7
Pretzels	16	Honey	12
Snickers Bar®	18	Hummus	0
		Pizza, plain, parmesan cheese, tomato sauce	22

the trend will continue as you age. In 10 or 20 years, it's likely that you'll need to make other adjustments in your diet.

I've experienced such change firsthand at two pivotal times in my life. The first was 1994, shortly after my 50th birthday. At the time, a running friend of mine, a professor at Colorado State University in Fort Collins, Colorado, tried to convince me that I needed to eat fewer refined carbs and more vegetables, fruits, and animal products. I argued that as an endurance athlete, I needed lots of carbs to train and race well. After all, the scientific literature was clear on that at the time. He challenged me to try what he recommended for one month. So I took him up on it just to show him that he was wrong.

For most of the first three weeks of the new diet, I felt terrible, recovered slowly, and craved carbs constantly. I thought I was well on my way to proving my argument. Then in the fourth week, something unusual happened. I started feeling better, recovered from workouts much more quickly, and no longer thought about sweet and starchy foods all day long. My training went very well that week. So I decided to try it for a fifth week and to up the ante by increasing my training load by half. Whenever I had done that in the previous few years, I had been likely to get a sore throat or head cold. This time I didn't. So I stayed at it for another week and once again increased the training load. No health problems, and training went well.

My friend now had my attention. I wanted to understand what was happening. He explained that my immune system was probably weak due to inadequate intake of micronutrients that was corrected by eating more vitamin- and mineral-dense foods. I've been eating that way ever since. (By the way, my friend is Loren Cordain, PhD, with whom 10 years later I coauthored a book based on his research called *The Paleo Diet for Athletes*.)

So things change with age. The diet I had been eating throughout my 20s, 30s, and 40s no longer worked as well by the time I turned 50. And it wouldn't be the last time this happened to me.

My body weight and belly girth had stayed quite stable for about five decades, ever since I had been a senior in high school. At age 18 I weighed 154 pounds (70 kg). I know that for a fact because I wrestled in the 154-pound weight class that year and never had to make weight to compete. Then in my mid-60s I noticed that something was changing. I started to gain a little excess belly fat in the winter as my weight climbed to the high 150s. I would count calories and take off the weight by the start of the spring race season. At age 68, however, my weight went to 166, and my formerly flat belly was quite plump. It was time to do something besides count calories and put up with constant hunger in the spring. I decided to make another small change to my diet.

It just so happened that I had been reading about low-carb, high-fat diets as proposed by Dr. Timothy Noakes, the author of *The Lore of Running* and other books. I've always respected his opinions and so decided to modify my diet a bit as he suggested to see what happened. That winter I cut back on almost all of the five or so servings of fruit I ate daily—about my only rich source of carbs other than sports drinks used while training—and began to eat more high-fat foods such as avocado, coconut cream and milk, nuts, nut butters, bacon, eggs, olive oil, and fish. The only fats I avoided were the human-made trans fats and omega-6 oils found mostly in junk foods.

What happened? Over the next 12 weeks my weight dropped back down to 154, and the belly fat was gone. The best part was that I never counted calories and always ate until satisfied. Once again I had changed my diet some 18 years after the first big transformation. Now, at age 70, I continue to eat as I learned to do at two different times in my life.

This is not to say that you need to make such changes. As I said earlier, nutrition is a very individualized science. It depends largely on your genetic makeup. What's right for one athlete isn't necessarily right for all. Instead, the lesson is that you may need to experiment with your diet to see what happens.

Recommendations for Change

If you answered yes to any of the above diet-related questions, it's time to consider altering your diet to make positive changes for your health and athletic performance. What changes should you make? Where should you start? These are very difficult questions to answer with any degree of certainty, given how individualized nutrition is. About the best we can do is to look at generally accepted solutions relative to what we know about diet and aging from research. The starting point is likely to be your protein intake, as it has been shown that there is an increased need for protein in older folks.[26]

I've mentioned the benefits of protein several times in previous chapters. Of course, I don't know exactly what you eat and how much protein you get in a day. You may be doing great in this regard. But for most aging athletes, it's probably a good idea to increase protein intake. Even if accumulating body fat isn't a problem, it's still a good idea to eat more animal products, the food type richest in protein and most absorbable by the body. The current U.S. Department of Agriculture recommended daily protein intake for adults is between 0.66 and 0.80 grams per kilogram of body weight.[27] Converting that to ounces and pounds means eating 0.023 to 0.028 ounces of protein per pound of body weight per day. For example, if you weigh 154 pounds, that calls for eating about 3.5 to 4.3 servings of roasted chicken breast in a day (a standard 3-ounce serving of chicken breast contains about 1 ounce of protein). For a 121-pound woman, it works out to about 2.8 to 3.4 servings of chicken breast daily. (Of course, you're unlikely to eat just one type of food to get your daily protein.)

More recent research, however, using a more precise way to measure the body's use of protein, strongly suggests that we need more as we age—0.93 to 1.2 g/kg/day, or 0.032 to 0.042 ounces per pound of body weight.[28] For a 154-pound man, that's 4.9 to 6.5 servings of chicken breast daily. For our 121-pound woman, it's 3.9 to 5.1 servings. That's a sizable increase of 40 to 50 percent more protein per day than previously recommended—and a lot of chicken breast. You're likely not eating anywhere near that amount now. You may not even be getting the much lower USDA recommended daily intake. That's why I suggest that you strongly consider eating more animal products. Table 8.2 lists the amounts of protein in a standard serving of common foods.

Athletes generally get most of their protein in the evening meal, as they are often focused on carbohydrate-rich foods throughout the day. But since only a small amount of protein can be processed by the body following a meal, if you eat most of it at dinner, which is likely to be about one serving, then much of it is unused by the body.[29] You'd be much better off spreading out your protein consumption, with three or four servings in a day. That means eating more animal products for breakfast and lunch than you may eat now and perhaps including a protein snack sometime during the day as well.

If you conclude that it is a good idea to eat more protein, you will need to remove something from your diet to keep from swelling the calorie intake. That leaves carbs and fat. I'd suggest replacing some of your carb intake with protein since carbohydrate plays no role in the health needs of people at any age and is more likely to add to belly size. You can live—in fact, thrive—on little or no carbohydrate. There is no carb requirement for health as there is for protein and fat. You may eat a prodigious amount of such foods now primarily because they taste good and help to fuel your training and racing. In fact, one study found that healthy elderly men (nonathletes) had a reduced capacity for producing energy from carbs and an increased capacity for using fat for fuel.[30] It's likely that this also applies to athletes and, in fact, may prove to be a good thing.

There are a couple of other upsides to eating protein. One big benefit for weight control is that of the three food types—protein, fat, and carbohydrate—protein is the most satiating.[31] That means that after a protein-rich meal, you're not likely to be hungry again for some time. You're satisfied. You're likely to eat less food overall, which may in turn lead to a loss of body fat over time.[32]

Another protein-eating benefit lies in its anabolic effect—it helps to build muscle with advancing age, especially for active athletes lifting weights, both men and women.[33] The body is in a constant state of rebuilding its muscles, and strength training accelerates that process. Only a small amount of muscle is replaced daily, but over the course of a few

TABLE 8.2. **Protein Content of Standard Servings of 23 Common Foods**

FOOD (serving size)	OUNCES OF PROTEIN PER SERVING	FOOD (serving size)	OUNCES OF PROTEIN PER SERVING
Chicken breast, roasted (3 oz)	0.95	Cheddar cheese (1 ounce)	0.25
Turkey, roasted, white meat (2 pieces)	0.88	Walnuts (1 ounce)	0.25
Hamburger (4 oz)	0.88	Bagel, plain (1)	0.25
Tuna, canned (3 oz)	0.85	Spaghetti, cooked (1 cup)	0.25
Steak, sirloin, broiled (3 oz)	0.81	Special K cereal (1 oz)	0.21
Pizza, cheese (1 slice)	0.53	Baked potato (1)	0.18
Kidney beans, red (1 cup)	0.53	Ice cream (1 cup)	0.18
		Peanut butter (1 tbsp)	0.18
Eggs, cooked (2)	0.42	Rice, brown (1 cup)	0.18
Lima beans (1 cup)	0.42	Whole-wheat bread (1 slice)	0.10
Yogurt, low-fat with fruit (8 oz)	0.35		
		Orange juice (1 cup)	0.07
Milk, skim (1 cup)	0.32	Apple (1)	0.0

weeks all of your muscles are replaced. To keep up with this rebuilding project, amino acids, the building blocks of protein, are needed.

Even simply eating protein stimulates the body to start rebuilding muscle. But as mentioned earlier, if your digestive system is overwhelmed with protein in a single meal, the excess will be mostly burned for immediate energy needs. Instead, you should distribute your protein consumption fairly evenly throughout the day.

When it comes to training, the time to take in protein is immediately following a workout.[34] The research is a bit equivocal on what "immediate" means. I'd suggest eating recovery food within an hour of finishing.

About three-quarters of an ounce of protein is adequate after lifting weights or doing other strenuous workouts (see Table 8.2). That's roughly a serving of chicken salad, a tuna-fish sandwich, 2 boiled eggs, or 3 ounces of cheese.

Other than eating adequate protein, another recommendation you should consider is removing junk food from your diet. That means cutting back on highly processed "artificial" foods—stuff your grandparents could never have eaten. If it comes in a plastic package, a bag, or a box, you should be highly suspicious that it's junk. These foods are typically high in both sugar and trans fats. Taken separately, sugar and trans fats are of high concern for your health. Combined, they are not only unhealthy but also highly likely to produce an increase in belly fat. Foods high in both sugar and fat have been shown to be the most fattening of all.[35] In the high-sugar-only category, sweetened beverages, such as soft drinks and fruit juices, are the most body-fat producing.

Training

Even serious endurance athletes gain body fat as they grow older. It happens to nearly all of us. Remember Michael Pollock's classic 10-year study of male elite runners from Chapter 1?[36] You may recall that some of them stopped racing and shifted their training from high intensity to long, slow distance. Over 10 years, that group added 15 percent more body fat to what they had a decade earlier. Even those who continued with high-intensity training and racing added fat—13 percent more. It appears that high-intensity training accounted for about 3 pounds less fat on average. That may not sound like a lot, but 3 pounds is roughly 36 seconds in a 10K running race or 6 watts of additional power needed to climb a hill on a bike.

That can easily make the difference between standing on the podium or watching the awards ceremony from the crowd.

We've been led to believe that long, slow distance is the way to go when it comes to controlling body fat. Very low heart rate training is often referred to as the "fat-burning zone." This is another case of a myth that refuses to go away. Low-intensity, slow exercise does *not* burn more calories or more fat than does high-intensity, fast-paced exercise. Nor do you lose more weight from going slow. It's actually just the opposite.

In a classic study on this topic, researchers at Laval University in Quebec, Canada, had one group of subjects, both men and women, exercise at a low intensity for 20 weeks.[37] Another group of men and women did high-intensity intervals (15 x 90-second sprints at 60–70 percent of maximum power) for 15 weeks. The low-intensity group burned a total of 28,757 kilocalories, while the high-intensity group burned 13,829. Sounds like I'm wrong, huh?

But guess what happened? The high-intensity group had much greater reductions in skin-fold measurements using the caliper fat-measuring technique. This was the result of increased fat burning during periods of rest *between* training sessions. In other words, the high-intensity group members significantly increased their metabolisms for the remainder of each exercise day to a much greater extent than the low-intensity exercisers did. That is, the high-intensity training produced significant increases in the enzymes that burn fat for fuel. The low-intensity group had no changes in these enzymes. In fact, they experienced a loss of enzymes over 20 weeks.

Note that the intensity levels for these two groups were extremely different. Heart rate zone 1, favored by the low-intensity group, is so easy that you wonder whether you are doing anything of value for your fitness.

On the other hand, the high-intensity level for its corresponding group was very high. It would be a mental challenge to do this workout several times a week for 15 weeks. As described in Chapter 6, however, you need a mix of different intensities in your training, including slow and easy recovery sessions following high-intensity intervals.

The bottom line is that high-intensity training is much more likely to result in the loss of excess flab than is long, slow distance done in the mythical "fat-burning zone." Hard workouts not only promote the production of the anabolic hormones you've read so much about here but also simply burn more calories over the course of your day. This dovetails very nicely with what you've read in the previous chapters about the benefits of aerobic-capacity and lactate-threshold interval sessions for performance, especially when combined with high-load strength training. High intensity is beneficial for both body composition and race results. Don't abandon it in a misguided attempt to lose body fat by doing only long, slow distance.

Menopause

Science still has a lot to learn about the human body. That's especially true when it comes to menopause and the aging female athlete. On the related topic of bone mineral density, there is no question that serious training is beneficial. Exercise, especially bone-loading exercise such as running and weight lifting, has been shown to be quite beneficial in keeping osteoporosis at bay while promoting the preservation of muscle with advancing age.[38] Science is less clear on the combined topic of body fat, age, and menopause. There's also general agreement that in the years during and after menopause, women are prone to lose muscle mass while gaining abdominal fat.[39]

How about shifts in body composition toward fat accumulation? What do we know about that from sport science? Interestingly, some research

GALE
BERNHARDT

Menopause

Experts consider menopause to have occurred after a woman experi-ences one year without menstruation. The average age for meno-pause is 51. Many women look forward to menopause because there is no more dealing with the messiness, inconvenience, and unpredictability of monthly periods.

Unfortunately, the five or so years leading up to menopause, defined as perimenopause, is often the beginning of a long list of frustrating symptoms for many women. Typical symptoms include hot flashes, night sweats, moodiness, insomnia, and headaches.

The most common symptom is the hot flash, which often begins with a sensation of pressure in the head quickly followed by a feeling of heat flushing through the body. Some women will experience hot flashes multiple times per day, several days per week. The most exasperating symptoms are the nighttime hot flashes and sheet-drenching sweats that disturb an otherwise good night of rest. Athletes who experience hot flashes and night sweats cannot recover from daily living, let alone training, because they cannot get a full night of sleep for days, some-times weeks, at a time.

For some women, the symptoms of perimenopause continue into postmenopause, or the period of time that is over one year after the cessation of menstruation. Usually postmenopausal symptoms are less severe. If you happen to be one of the women who has these pesky symptoms, often for 5 to 10-plus years, it is obviously exasperating.

Not every woman experiences extreme or even average symptoms. My menopause age was 52, and at the writing of this book, I am 55. Compared with some women I know, my symptoms were extremely minor. I had a few hot flashes in the perimenopausal years, and those were typically associated with menstrual cycles, but not all cycles. »

Continued

In hindsight, I estimate that I had fewer than six hot flashes in any single year.

I will admit to occasional (in my opinion) "crabby-pants" mood swings. I know that for some women, a constant feeling of grumpiness is common. I suspect this is in a large part a result of very-low-quality sleep and the vexing inability to predict when the "power surge" of a hot flash will attack.

I didn't use any special creams, herbs, or prescription medicines and made no special doctor visits to address the symptoms. I didn't modify training at all, before or after menopause, due to "female issues." There were certainly some low-energy days, but these could easily be attributed to other things going on in my life.

As menopause goes, I'm not sure why I got off so easy, but I'll take it. It is possible that some combination of genetics, lifestyle, diet, stress management, and exercise patterns caused the low level of menopausal issues. One of my good friends also got off easy, so I am not a solo example.

For those reading this book and heading into menopause, my message is that not everyone experiences debilitating perimenopause, menopause, and postmenopause symptoms. I hope that, like me, you are one of the fortunate ones.

has found no cause-and-effect relationship between menopause and increases in body fat.[40] But I've talked with many female athletes who tell me something different. Most of the research on this topic supports their opinion. According to most of the limited studies, there is at least a strong association between menopause and increase in body fat, which suggests—but of course does not prove—cause.[41] So the jury is still out. If menopause is eventually shown to cause fat accumulation, especially in the abdominal area, there is little that can be done about it other than hormone replacement therapy, which is not as effective as high-intensity training for controlling body composition.[42] Hormone replacement therapy is also fraught with its own health implications.[43]

Medications

Another possible cause of an aging athlete's increasing weight and waist girth is prescription drugs. If you experience a change in body fat after starting a medication or switching to a new one, then suspecting the drug is warranted. Of course, the physical change may be so slow in occurring that it's hard to pinpoint when it started and therefore what the culprit is. Nevertheless, any pills or pharmacological treatments you are receiving should be considered when you are measurably gaining fat, especially if your eating habits and training have not changed. Prescription drugs have frequently been shown to result in weight gain, but not all people respond to a given drug by gaining weight. Some may even lose weight.[44] To further complicate things, the weight gain could be the result of water retention rather than added body fat. Your increased corpulence could also result from a drug-stimulated increase in appetite or fatigue resulting in a lower level of training.

Drugs that are known to often cause weight gain are those used in the treatment of heart conditions such as angina, high blood pressure, and arrhythmias; asthma; arthritis; mood disorders; neurological disorders; diabetes; migraine headaches; epilepsy; cancer; and a host of other miscellaneous conditions, including allergies and hormone replacement therapies.[45]

The place to start when you think that your meds may be the root cause is with your doctor, who may prescribe a different drug or a lower dosage. Never stop taking a prescribed drug or change the dose without talking with your doctor first.

Body Fat

The take-home message from this chapter is that your percentage of body fat relative to lean tissue is likely to increase as you get older. This is almost certainly due to a slowing of your metabolism.[46] As we saw earlier, a common misconception is that muscle turns into fat as you age. For many, that seems to make sense because fat does indeed increase in the very places that used to be firm and muscular. But that's not how it happens. Muscle slowly withers away with disuse while fat takes up residence. These are separate events that just happen to occur at about the same time.

The best way I've found to fight back is through regular vigorous exercise. High-intensity workouts stimulate the production of anabolic hormones, such as growth hormone and testosterone, which raise your body's metabolism and cut fat accumulation. Long, slow distance workouts are not nearly as effective at accomplishing this; high-intensity training, including heavy-load strength training, is the way to go. Unfortunately, the low-intensity, fat-burning myth has been around for such a long time that even professional coaches and trainers, who should know better, keep it going. Workouts such as aerobic-capacity and lactate-threshold intervals are likely to produce far greater reductions in body fat while also greatly contributing to performance in aging athletes.

As a senior athlete, you need to be cautious about the introduction of intervals and weight lifting to your training in order to avoid injuries. But when safely practiced, this regimen is the surest available method for trimming unwanted fat, staying strong, and staying competitive throughout your sports career.

Epilogue

There's no doubt that athletic performance declines with age. It's inevitable. You're undoubtedly experiencing this yourself. The decline is usually quite noticeable by age 50 and, according to research, appears to take a rather severe plunge around 70.

Take heart, however: Some of this reported performance loss later in life may be merely the result of aging statistics. There are relatively few athletes over the age of 70 who have spent most of their lives training and competing at a high level. Most came to sport late in life and have not had many age peers with whom to compete. In light of this, rapid decline in those who have already had their 70th birthday is to be expected. But with the leading edge of the baby-boomer generation reaching their late 60s as this book is being written, I fully expect to see statistical changes in the expected decline after 70. If you count yourself among this group, then you are part of the most athletic and performance-focused generation in history. I believe you will rewrite the numbers in such a way that we may soon find that the rate of decline for athletes in their eighth decade of life is no greater than it was in the previous 10 years.

That doesn't mean age isn't an issue. While the rate at which it occurs may be open for interpretation, performance in endurance sports does indeed decline due to aging. But sports scientists are increasingly coming to the conclusion that much of the loss, if not most of it, is the result of changes in lifestyle and training. Age by itself does not account for all of the decline. If that is indeed true, what can you do to minimize the losses?

Throughout this book I've suggested training routines involving high-intensity training at or near your aerobic capacity, heavy-load strength training, the possible modification of your periodized training routine, and frequent and regular testing of progress. You've also read about other lifestyle factors that influence high performance such as diet, sleep, recovery methods, and body composition. If you want to perform at a higher level, I'm certain that the adoption of some of the training and lifestyle factors you've read about in the previous chapters will help you succeed.

Of course, I realize that not everyone seeks high performance or can achieve it. There are three common reasons for not making changes in one's lifestyle and training: motivation, injury, and health.

Many older athletes simply enjoy doing their daily easy workout and don't want to change either their training routine or lifestyle. Exercise for such athletes has become as common as eating and sleeping, which also seem to be going quite well. There's nothing wrong with that. Regular, easy exercise coupled with a healthy diet and adequate sleep certainly promotes a long and active life. Keep it up!

On the other hand, you may want to compete again at a high level but are held back from doing high-intensity exercise by the risk of injury. Unfortunately, that's quite common for older athletes, especially runners. This is perhaps the most challenging situation experienced by serious senior athletes. There is no easy solution. But there may be ways to resolve the challenge.

The starting point is to find the reason for your susceptibility to physical breakdown and work to eliminate it. When I was coaching full time (I'm now retired from training athletes), I started all of my athletes' seasons by taking them to a physical therapist who works primarily with athletes. Each client got a head-to-toe exam with the purpose of discovering his or her potential areas for injury. Every athlete was found to have some likely area for breakdown—a tendon, joint, muscle, or something else. And the older he or she was, the more potential injury sites were typically found. The therapist would then design a personalized treatment plan to reduce and perhaps prevent the occurrence of injury. The plan usually included functional strength work, range-of-motion exercises, equipment change, and modified training routines. The athlete was also given a progression plan—how quickly to increase the stress for each exercise. We learned what to watch throughout the season for signs that indicated a need to dial back training. We also learned how to care for a niggling injury in the very early stages to prevent it from interrupting training. As a coach, my role was to see to the implementation while monitoring the injury-prevention plan along with the athlete.

You can do the same. Through your coach, your athletic club, or your primary physician, seek out the counsel of an experienced physical therapist. Describe your exercise and competition goals, itemize your former injuries, and get a thorough evaluation of your physical condition. An injury-free season of fulfilling competition may be closer than you think.

There also may be reasons that athletes can't train with high intensity due to health conditions or medications they are on. If this is the case, you need to closely follow your doctor's instructions, of course, but you also should seek additional medical opinions. Read everything you can find on the topic with the goal of becoming an expert on your condition. And ask your doctor challenging questions. This is not to say that you should disregard what your doctor tells you so that you can exercise more intensely. My point is that you need to be in control. Your health is your responsibility, not your doctor's. By being highly proactive, you're more likely to improve your health and may eventually return to a higher level of training. Don't give up.

As I was doing the research for this book it became apparent to me that I was in the first group described earlier. My training and lifestyle were slowly shifting toward comfort and somewhat easier workouts. I had stopped lifting weights, and my training intensity had been steadily declining over the past couple of years. While I watched my diet and body composition closely, I was getting less sleep than I had a few years prior. No wonder my performance was trending the wrong way.

You may recall from the Prologue that this book started out as my personal project to avoid such losses. I wanted to read as much aging research as I could find to learn how to stave off the ravages of growing older. I anticipated a substantial decline in performance sometime after my 70th birthday. Looking back now with the clarity of time on my side, I realize that the decline actually started a couple of years earlier, when I was 68. In a bike race that spring, I was dropped by the small lead group on a climb in the mountains outside Boulder, Colorado. I had never been dropped in a race before. At the time I chalked up the poor performance to my recent arrival in the thin mountain air of Colorado, which is a mile above my home in Scottsdale, Arizona. But altitude may not have been the reason at all.

Over the next year other small performance-related changes occurred. The most notable was a drop in my measured power output on the bike. It wasn't a huge difference, but my power was now somewhat lower than the normal winter variations that always occurred. And this time the drop was unique because it did not return to its previously high summer levels that year.

That summer before my 70th birthday, I started the research-reading project. As a result of digging through the research for the common causes of performance decline with aging, I became aware of the importance of aerobic capacity and strength training. The critical workouts were easy once I understood the likely problems. I subsequently developed a nine-day training cycle to allow for more rest between such hard workouts. The nine-day week significantly improved the overall quality of my training. As a result of reading the research, I also came to fully grasp the importance of sleep duration with age. Mine had been dropping in the past few years as I cut back on sleep in order to get more done each day.

In early November, just shy of two months prior to my Big Seven-Zero Day, I gradually incorporated all of these changes into my training and lifestyle. I did aerobic-capacity and lactate-threshold intervals, lifted heavy weights, changed my periodization routine to a nine-day platform, and got considerably more sleep. And the new routine began to show results. By the end of January, a full month after my 70th birthday, my power, which is one of the best indicators of cycling performance, had risen by 7 percent in testing. That's the biggest increase I had ever seen in such a short time. All of the changes seemed to be paying off.

Then, four days after that test, it all came crashing down—literally.

A month after my dreaded birthday, I crashed on a recovery bike workout when an exceptionally strong gust of wind blew me into a curb that projected into the bike lane on a descent. I broke seven bones and had a concussion. Six days later I was out of the hospital and back home when my doctor, a former triathlon client, discovered that I had developed blood clots in my legs and lungs. He put me on a blood-thinning medication for six months.

As I write this, I still have another month of the drug regimen remaining. While I returned to riding three weeks after the crash, I confess that

I have not made much progress. There is some evidence that the medication I'm taking may affect red-blood-cell production, reducing the blood's capacity for carrying oxygen to the muscles. Regardless, I've had a gigantic loss of power and endurance in training. So much for my race plans for this season. Now my focus is just on health and exercise enjoyment. How quickly things can change!

Temporary setbacks are common in sport. I hope I'll return to a normal life at about the time this book is published and be back to racing again after my 71st birthday. Along the way I'll certainly return to doing all of the senior athlete performance enhancers I've described in these pages. I'm confident they work. I'd enjoy hearing of your experiences with them in your quest to improve performance. Please e-mail me with how you are doing at jfriel@trainingbible.com. I look forward to hearing from you.

Acknowledgments

I'm very fortunate to have a friend such as Bill Cofer. We've been like brothers since we first met by chance in August 1971, when he sat down next to me at a meeting. We've grown old together, and over 40 years, I've come to trust Bill's thoughts and suggestions. We have much in common. He's an endurance athlete who is only five years younger than I. He's also smart—much smarter than I, I've found. So I asked him to read the chapters of this book as I wrote them and tell me what he thought. He did much more than that; he also read the research studies on which I based much of this book. And there were many. Bill, once again you've proven to be a great friend and a wise man. I owe you a great deal. Thanks, brother!

I also owe a great deal to the distinguished group of athletes and doctors, all over the age of 50, who contributed their wisdom and experiences to this book: Mark Allen; Gale Bernhardt; Amby Burfoot; Larry Creswell, MD; John Howard; Tim Noakes, MD; Ned Overend; John Post, MD; Andy Pruitt, EdD; and Lisa Rainsberger. Their insights added depth to many topics that I only touch on.

On the production side I want to thank Publisher Ted Costantino at VeloPress for once again trusting me to write a book that not only is meaningful for the reader but will add value to the VeloPress catalog. Ted was a tremendous help in focusing the content up front, and he did the initial edit. Connie Oehring copyedited the manuscript and asked good questions about what I *intended* to say. Thanks, Connie!

Finally, I want to thank the hundreds of senior athletes who have been so kind in telling me about their training, race performances, and lifestyles over the years. Many of you have proven to be great personal mentors while also asking me questions that more sharply focused my thinking about the aging process. I hope you find something of value for your athletic goals in this book.

Workout Guidelines for Senior Athletes

The Aerobic-Capacity Workout

High-intensity training, especially aerobic-capacity intervals, will boost your VO_2max (see Chapter 6 for more details). Here are the details of how to design the components of an aerobic-capacity interval session. As always, you should precede your interval session with a warm-up of sufficient duration and intensity to elevate your heart rate and breathing. This workout may also be done as fartlek.

1. Interval duration. The length of the interval may be as short as 30 seconds or as long as 3 minutes. If you haven't done such challenging workouts in several years—or even several months—start with shorter durations such as 30 to 60 seconds.

2. Recovery duration. The easy recovery time between the intervals should be the same duration as the preceding interval. So if you just finished a 30-second interval, recover for 30 seconds. "Recover" in this case means to go very easily.

3. Intensity. There are many ways to determine intensity. A lab test is likely to be the most accurate. But the simplest and least expensive test is to do a 5-minute, all-out time trial. You can do this by yourself or with a training partner for motivation. The appropriate intensity for your intervals is either your average speed or your average power for the full 5 minutes. To determine speed, do the self-test on a measured course, such as a track for runners or a known course for cyclists, or by using an indoor training device such as an ergometer or a treadmill. For some sports, measuring speed outdoors may be greatly affected by wind and hills, so take those variables into account. For power, use a power meter.

4. Workout duration. Again, if you haven't done a high-intensity workout in some time, such as a few months or more, then do only a combined interval duration of 5 minutes for the initial workout. That would work out to something such as 10 × 30 seconds or 5 × 60 seconds. As your training progresses over several weeks, increase the workout duration gradually until you are doing a total of about 15 minutes of high-intensity intervals— something such as 7 × 2 minutes or 5 × 3 minutes. Progress slowly and gradually over several weeks.

5. Frequency. How often should you do a high-intensity interval session? The answer has to do with how fast you recover, which can vary considerably among athletes. Some will be able to do another hard session after two or three days of recovery. Others may need an entire week between interval sessions. If unsure, start with one such session in seven days. Judge how you feel when training for the next few days, and make frequency adjustments accordingly.

6. Use caution. High-intensity workouts are risky due to the effort and strain placed on muscles, tendons, and joints. Approach these workouts with caution, especially regarding the level of intensity. If you haven't done such training in a long time, start with intervals that correspond to your training plan's "hard" zone (about 15 on the Borg RPE scale or 4 in my zone system; see Appendix C for more details).

The Lactate-Threshold Workout

This interval session will boost your lactate-threshold speed or power (see Chapter 6 for more details). Following are details of how to design the lactate-threshold interval session. As always, you should precede the interval session by a warm-up of sufficient duration and intensity to elevate your heart rate and breathing.

1. Interval duration. See Table 6.1, repeated here as Table A.1 (next page).

2. Recovery duration. See Table A.1.

3. Intensity. This may be determined with a lab test or a 20-minute time trial. If you are doing a time trial, subtract 5 percent from your speed or power to determine intensity level for the lactate-threshold workout. You can also use your average heart rate minus 5 percent for the entire 20-minute time trial to determine lactate-threshold heart rate. Subtracting another 5 percent produces a lactate-threshold heart rate training zone that is 5 to 10 percent lower than the average heart rate for the 20-minute time trial. If you intend to gauge intensity using perceived exertion, the proper intensity would be 6 or 7 on a 1-to-10 scale.

TABLE A.1. **Suggested Training Details for High-, Moderate-, and Low-Dose Workouts**

WORKOUT TYPE	HIGH DOSE	MODERATE DOSE	LOW DOSE
Aerobic-capacity intervals Intensity at or slightly below VO₂max speed/power/ perceived exertion	5 × 2.5 min (2.5 min recoveries) 5 × 3 min (3 min recoveries)	6 × 1.5 min (1.5 min recoveries) 5 × 2 min (2 min recoveries)	10 × 30 sec (30 sec recoveries) 7 × 1 min (1 min recoveries)
Lactate-threshold intervals Intensity: 90–95% of LTHR* or 88–93% of FTP** speed/power.	3 × 12 min (3 min 15 sec recoveries) 2 × 20 min (5 min recoveries)	3 × 8 min (2.5 min recoveries) 3 × 10 min (3 min recoveries)	3 × 5 min (90 sec recoveries) 3 × 6 min (2 min recoveries)
Aerobic threshold Intensity: continuous and steady at about 30 bpm < LTHR* ± 2 bpm. Duration: dependent on goal event.	2–4 hr	1–2 hr	30 min–1 hr
Weight lifting Simulate the movements of your sport with full recoveries after each set. Low reps mean high loads.	7–9 reps 3–6 reps	13–15 reps 10–12 reps	20–30 reps 16–19 reps

* Lactate-threshold heart rate; ** Functional Threshold Power
Note: Each workout is preceded by a warm-up and followed by a cooldown.

4. Workout duration. This session needs to be only as long as the time needed for the warm-up, the intervals, and the cooldown. That would typically cause it to take at least an hour. For some sports, especially those with events that last longer than 2 hours, it may be advantageous to extend the warm-up and cooldown to increase your endurance capacity.

5. Frequency. Since this session is somewhat less stressful than aerobic-capacity intervals, it can typically be done more frequently. It's common for younger senior athletes to be able to do this workout twice in a seven- to nine-day period, but older seniors are probably best advised to do it only once in the same time frame.

6. Use caution. The stress on soft tissues is moderate in this workout, but it's certainly greater than that of long, slow distance training. If you haven't done a workout like this recently, then use caution in determining how great the dose will be and how frequently you will do it.

The Aerobic-Threshold Workout

This is a steady-state session intended to improve your aerobic threshold speed or power along with your capability for using fat as your primary fuel source (see Chapter 6 for more details). This session should be preceded by a short warm-up to elevate your heart rate into a light endurance workout zone (about 10 on the Borg RPE scale or zone 2 in my system; see Appendix C for more details).

1. Duration. See Table A.1.

2. Recovery duration. See Table A.1.

3. Intensity. This may be determined by a lab test. For a rough estimate, subtract 30 beats per minute from your lactate-threshold heart rate, then add and subtract 2 bpm from that heart rate to create a 5-bpm zone. For example, if your lactate-threshold heart rate is 150 bpm, subtracting 30 results in an estimated heart rate of 120. Adding and subtracting 2 produces a heart rate range of 118 to 122.

TABLE A.2. **Duration of Aerobic-Threshold Workout Based on Goal Event's Duration**

Duration of goal event	>4 hr	2–4 hr	<2 hr
Aerobic-threshold workout duration	2–4 hr	1–2 hr	30 min–1 hr

4. Workout duration. Duration should be 30 minutes to 4 hours. See Table 6.2, repeated here as Table A.2, for the details of your specific event needs.

5. Frequency. This is a low-stress workout that can be done as often as you see fit.

6. Use caution. While the workout may be low stress, that doesn't mean it's no stress. You will probably find that you are a bit tired the day after such a session. Doing this workout too frequently will result in accumulating a significant amount of fatigue. With fatigue comes the threat of injury or breakdown for other reasons. Continue to be cautious.

The Strength Training Workout

The following are suggestions for how to design a strength training program if you haven't lifted weights in years, or even a few months (see Chapter 6 for more details). I highly recommend that you consult a personal trainer or coach who knows your sport. Warm up with aerobic exercise such as riding a stationary bike or running slowly on a treadmill.

1. Frequency. Lift weights once or twice per week. If you are new to strength training, or if you haven't done it in a long time, start with one session per week. After two or three sessions in as many weeks, increase your frequency to two strength sessions in a week with three or four days between them.

2. Exercises. Choose exercises that are specific to your sport. For example, a runner should build strength in the primary muscles that are used in running—the calf, thigh, and butt. If you are unsure which muscles need strength building for your sport or the proper, sport-specific exercises for those muscles, ask for help from a personal trainer at your gym or a coach who understands your sport. Triathletes, road cyclists, and mountain bikers will find complete, sport-specific strength programs in my books *The Triathlete's Training Bible, The Cyclist's Training Bible,* and *The Mountain Biker's Training Bible.*

3. Sets. Do two or three sets in a workout. A "set" is a grouping of continuous repetitions (reps) with a given load. Three sets of 20 reps would be written as "3 × 20."

4. Loads. Start with loads you can easily manage, and increase them gradually. If you are getting back into strength training after a few years or even just a few weeks of weight lifting inactivity, be very cautious. Start with ridiculously easy loads—body weight or an empty barbell is usually adequate at first, especially as you are mastering a particular exercise (you need to master the lifting technique before you add weight). Gradually add weight until you can manage to do only about 20 reps in a set. Then over the course of several sessions, increase the loads until you can manage about 15 reps in a set. After several sessions at 15 reps, slowly increase the loads to the point where you can manage about 10 reps per set. The final step is about 3 to 9 reps per set with relatively heavy loads. This gradual and steady progression should keep you uninjured while making great gains in strength. Plan on this progression taking 8 weeks or more. After completing 6 to 8 sessions of 3 to 9 reps per set, it's time to move into a maintenance mode.

5. Recovery. Fully recover after each set. After the weight is set down following the last rep in each set, relax and allow the fatigued muscles to recover for 2 to 3 minutes, much as if you were doing intervals, before starting the next set or exercise.

6. Core strength. Consider including core strengthening exercises in your program. The core muscles are those in your trunk that primarily support your spine and also the shoulders and pelvis. Some athletes have poor core strength. This often is evident in their inability to maintain good full-body posture while making the movements of their sport.

Field Tests for Senior Athletes

Aerobic-Threshold Test

In Chapter 4 I introduced the idea of comparing output (speed, pace, or power) with input (effort or heart rate) to find something called the "Efficiency Factor" (EF). There it was suggested as a way of determining how your interval workouts are progressing. This same method is also useful in determining changes in aerobic fitness from week to week by measuring the EF of your aerobic threshold.

If you know your lactate-threshold heart rate based on a lab test or a 20-minute test (described below in the section titled "Lactate-Threshold Test"), subtract 30 beats per minute for a rough estimate of your aerobic threshold. For athletes using my heart rate zone system, that calculation will place your aerobic threshold around upper zone 1 or lower zone 2 (see Appendix C for details). Of course, you can get a much more accurate estimate of your aerobic threshold if you pay for a lab test.

Knowing this, all you need to gauge aerobic-threshold progress is to measure EF using your heart rate monitor along with either a stopwatch, a speed-and-distance device, or a power meter. Efficiency—how much effort or energy it takes to produce a speed or a power level—is one of the best indicators of fitness for endurance athletes. Let me refresh your memory on how to measure EF. Then we'll apply it to your aerobic threshold.

The starting point when measuring training progress is to control as many potential performance-affecting variables as possible. You need to gather lots of data, which means that you must record EF over the course of several workouts performed over several weeks. The sessions to be compared should be quite similar in terms of the course, duration, and especially intensity. Doing this test at your aerobic-threshold heart rate is the perfect intensity for measuring EF. For example, once a week do an aerobic-threshold workout on the same course, with the same warm-up, and at the same heart rate range (use your aerobic-threshold heart rate plus and minus 2 beats per minute) for the test portion.

The aerobic-threshold portion of the workout may take several minutes to a few hours to complete. How long depends on the event for which you are training. An Ironman triathlon and a 5K running race, while both endurance events, have nowhere near the same endurance demands, so the workouts will be of different durations.

TABLE B.1. **Example of Efficiency Factor Determination Using a Stopwatch or Speed-and-Distance Device**

Average heart rate (bpm)	125
Average speed (mph)	7.5 (to convert pace to speed, divide 60 by pace in minutes; e.g., an 8-minute pace is 60 ÷ 8 = 7.5 mph)
Average speed (yards/min)	220 (7.5 × 1,760 yards in a mile ÷ 60, the number of minutes in an hour)
Efficiency factor	1.76 (220 ÷ 125)

Note: The 3-mile test portion (following a warm-up) is done at the aerobic threshold with an average heart rate of 125 bpm.

TABLE B.2. **Example of Efficiency Factor Determination Using a Power Meter**

Average heart rate (bpm)	125
Normalized Power (watts)	150
Efficiency Factor	1.2 (150 ÷ 125)

Note: The 30-minute test portion (following a warm-up) is done at the aerobic threshold with an average heart rate of 125 bpm.

When done, divide your average speed (in yards per minute) or Normalized Power (if you are calculating with power; see my book *The Power Meter Handbook* for an explanation of this) for the test portion of the workout by your average heart rate for the same portion. Table 5.1, repeated here as Table B.1, provides an example of how to calculate EF using a stopwatch or a speed-and-distance device for runners, swimmers, and Nordic skiers. For cyclists or rowers using a power meter, see Table 5.2, repeated here as Table B.2, for an example.

Aerobic-Capacity Test

In Chapter 3 you read that your speed or power at aerobic capacity (VO_2max) can be maintained for about 5 minutes. That means you can self-conduct a field test to measure changes without having to go to a lab and pay for expensive testing using sophisticated equipment. I'd recommend testing your aerobic capacity every three to six weeks throughout the training season. It's simple, and it is a useful gauge of fitness.

Here's how to do the test if you are using a speed-and-distance device or a power meter. Following a warm-up, go as fast as you can on a standard course for 5 minutes. The course may be flat or have a continuous upgrade. It is best that it not be a rolling course with both uphill and downhill sections. If you are using a stopwatch because you don't have a speed-and-distance device or a power meter, you need to make only one slight change. Instead of using time as the fixed variable, you'll keep the distance constant. Measure a section of the course that you think will take about 5 minutes, and mark the start and finish points.

Whichever way you do it, use the same course every time you test. The first few times athletes do this test, they almost always start too fast. It's best to start slightly slower than you think is possible and speed up in the latter half.

This test is best done when rested and recovered from the previous several days of training. That means the best time to test is after a few days of rest and recovery (for details, see Chapter 6).

Of course, what you should see happen over time is that your speed or power for 5 minutes, or your time on a measured course, improves. This is a good indicator that fitness, especially aerobic capacity, is improving. That's one of the key markers of performance in senior athletes, as research has shown it to be the predictor of fitness that declines the fastest with aging.

Lactate-Threshold Test

This is quite similar to the 5-minute test except that it's longer. It serves as an indicator of how your lactate-threshold fitness, as described in Chapter 3, is progressing. Lactate-threshold fitness is considered the second most likely predictor of fitness to decline with aging.

Everything is the same as in the 5-minute test except that this one involves going fast for 20 minutes, or on a measured course that takes about 20 minutes. Also as before, do this test every three to six weeks following an R&R break from hard training. It's best that you use the same course every time you do the test, and the course should be either flat or slightly uphill. Don't use a course that has significant downhill sections. As with the 5-minute test, improved fitness is indicated by a greater average speed or higher power over 20 minutes, or by a faster time on a standard measured course that takes about 20 minutes to complete.

The 20-minute test may be used to estimate your Functional Threshold Power (FTPo) or Functional Threshold Pace (FTPa). For FTPo, subtract 5 percent from your Normalized Power for the test. For FTPa, convert pace to speed by dividing 60 by your average 1-mile pace for the test. Again, subtract 5 percent to estimate FTPa. In a similar manner you can get a good approximation of your lactate-threshold heart rate by subtracting 5 percent from your average heart rate for the 20 minutes.

$$\cdots$$

These two tests may be done within the same workout, or you can do them on separate days. If done the same day, do the 5-minute test first, with a long recovery following it before starting the 20-minute test. Of course, what you'd like to see is a greater speed or power, or a faster time indicating that fitness is improving.

The key principle in testing is: That which is measured improves. By observing and recording your EF in your training journal on a weekly basis and your aerobic-capacity and lactate-threshold test results every few weeks, you will be keenly aware of your training and how it is affecting your fitness. That means you can make training corrections whenever it becomes apparent that things aren't going as planned. You may, for example, find with testing that your EF is coming along quite well, but your aerobic capacity is not improving at all. That may lead you to make changes in your training to include more aerobic-capacity interval workouts. Without accurate feedback, you might not find out until race day, at which point it is impossible to improve.

Measuring Intensity

Throughout this book, I have referred to the use of training zones to ensure that you are either working hard enough to improve or going easy enough to recover (many athletes go too hard on recovery days, which makes monitoring intensity during recovery just as valuable as during workouts).

Due to the scope of this book, it isn't possible to cover training zones for every endurance sport. Instead, I have assumed that as a lifelong endurance athlete, you have probably been using a training zone system throughout your athletic career. I have further assumed that you will use that system to complete the workouts and plans presented here.

However, to make sure we are on the same page, it may be useful to review the various methods used to measure intensity. I've adapted the text that follows from the third edition of my book *The Triathlete's Training Bible*. You can find a more comprehensive explanation of training zones there, and you can find specific workout plans and training tables tied to training zones for swimming, cycling, and running in that book. For cycling only, zones and training tables are presented in *The Cyclist's Training Bible*.

...

How do you know which intensity zone you are in? Because heart rate monitors are now so common, endurance athletes have come to think of the heart as the best indicator of intensity. Such an exaggerated emphasis on heart rate has caused many to forget that it is not heart rate that limits performance in races and training. After all, fatigue occurs mostly in the muscles, not the cardiovascular system. The beating of the heart is merely one way to peek into the body to see what is happening.

At best, heart rate is an indirect measure of intensity, and not a very sensitive one. Other methods should also be used whenever possible to quantify how intensely you are exercising. Just like heart rate, though, each method has shortcomings. By employing two or more methods every time you work out, you will learn how to accurately gauge intensity and reap the desired training benefits.

Pace

In the early days of endurance sports such as running, cycling, and triathlon, training intensity was based primarily on pace. Pace is emphasized less now, which is too bad because it is an effective measure that can provide useful information. Pace is still, in fact, the best gauge of swimming intensity.

It used to be that if you wanted to run at a given pace there was only one way to do it. You would go to a measured course, such as a track, convert the goal pace into 400-meter or 200-meter splits, and start running. Of course, you wouldn't find out until you completed a split whether you were on pace or not. And then while running you'd have to do the math to figure out just how off target your pace was and how much to speed up or slow down. Experienced runners developed the ability to gauge exactly how fast they were going based on perceived exertion.

Fortunately, technology has made pace training more precise. A wristband GPS device can determine your position, pace, and distance using satellite technology. GPS, short for Global Positioning System, is accurate to within as little as 3 meters, depending on the device you use and how strong a signal it receives. (Civilian GPS used to be intentionally degraded to make it less accurate than military GPS, but that is no longer the case.)

Another useful device is the accelerometer. This electromechanical sensor measures movement changes—accelerations—to record pace and distance. For runners it comes with a small pod that fastens to a shoe. The accelerometer is built into the pod along with a small transmitter that wirelessly relays the data to a wristwatch where your pace and other information is displayed.

Some devices include other features as well, such as a heart rate monitor, and the capability to download the data to your computer for analysis. Neither a GPS nor an accelerometer is cheap, but prices vary considerably based on the features and functions included.

So which device is right for you? If you run in places where the sky is often blocked out by tall trees or buildings, then an accelerometer is the way to go. The accelerometer is also useful if you run frequently on treadmills. But if you tend to switch shoes for your runs, the GPS option is more convenient.

The key with using any such device for training is to think of it only as a tool to help you train more precisely. If you try to "beat" the device or spend all of your time looking at your wrist rather than paying attention to how you feel, it will detract from, rather than enhance, your running enjoyment and performance.

Rating of Perceived Exertion (RPE)

The experienced athlete has a well-developed ability to assess level of exertion based strictly on sensations emanating from the body's many systems. Perceived exertion is one of the best indicators of intensity, and it is used by all athletes, whether they are aware of it or not. In fact, after years of training, many pros don't even wear heart rate monitors while training and instead rely on a combination of pace and perceived exertion.

Perceived exertion is quantifiable using the Borg Rating of Perceived Exertion (RPE) scale, which scientists frequently use to determine the levels their test subjects reach. Many coaches and athletes also rely on RPE as the supreme gauge of effort. Borg's RPE is applicable to any sport. It's based on a scale of 6 to 20, with 6 representing no exertion at all and 20 signifying a maximum, all-out effort with absolutely nothing held in reserve. The scale of 6 to 20 was chosen because this range corresponds to the heart rates experienced by a moderately fit, young to middle-aged person, as each number is 10 percent of a typical heart rate for that perceived exertion. In other words, a score of 6 (resting) should parallel a heart rate of about 60 beats per minute, and 20 (maximum) should indicate a pulse of 200. In reality, these numbers seldom equate so nicely, since heart rates vary considerably at different exertion levels for different individuals.

(By the way, even though the science says that we lose 1 beat per minute of maximum heart rate every year, that is just a guess, and it may not be true for readers of this book. For example, my maximum heart rate has not changed since 1983, when I got my first heart rate monitor. I suspect that is likely to be true for you as well if you have trained at a high level for decades.)

To use the Borg RPE scale, give an honest appraisal of the feeling of exertion you experience while working out, and assign it a number on the scale. As you increase or decrease the pace, your RPE will also change, reflecting greater or lesser stress. The main problem athletes encounter

TABLE C.1. **Training Zone Rating System and Its Correlation with the Borg RPE Scale**

TRAINING ZONE	DESCRIPTION	BORG RPE SCALE	DESCRIPTION
1	Recovery	6	
		7	Very, very light
		8	
2	Extensive endurance	9	Very light
		10	
		11	Fairly light
3	Intensive endurance	12	
		13	Somewhat hard
		14	
4	Threshold	15	Hard
5a	Muscular endurance	16	Harder
5b	Anaerobic endurance	17	Very hard
		18	
5c	Power	19	Very, very hard
		20	

when using RPE is their own tendency to underestimate their exertion level to appear tough or brave. Moral value judgments should not accompany effort assessments. It should be a cold, scientific endeavor.

I created a modified version of the Borg RPE scale to use with my athletes and in my Training Bibles. I simplified the scale to 1 through 5, with three subcategories for the 5 scale (5a, 5b, and 5c). Table C.1 shows the correspondence between the training zones I use and the Borg RPE scale.

Heart Rate

In the 1980s, the introduction of the wireless heart rate monitor brought a profound change to the way athletes in all endurance sports trained.

Since intensity could not be directly measured, volume was generally considered the key to race fitness. Using the monitor taught us that by varying intensity across a broad spectrum of heart rates, great benefits were possible. We learned how to improve recovery by using the monitor to slow down. The monitor also taught us that more intense workouts were often possible. The monitor allowed us to not only accurately determine intensity but also to measure progress and gauge effort in a long race.

The problem is that heart rate–based training has become so pervasive that athletes too often believe that heart rate is the determining factor in how they train and race. Too many have become slaves to their heart rate monitors and do not use other tools for measuring intensity as much as they could. Heart rate is but one window into how your body is doing. It may give you a better perspective on the exercising body, but this is not the only perspective that is worthwhile. Relying on it to the exclusion of all other measures of intensity can be as detrimental to your training as not having any gauge of effort at all.

When used intelligently, however, the heart rate monitor can improve fitness and race performance. Sometimes low motivation, high enthusiasm, competition, loss of focus, and poor judgment get in the way of smart training. In these instances the heart rate monitor is like having a coach along for the workout. With a good working knowledge of heart rate, skill in using other intensity measures, and a little common sense resulting from experience, you can use a monitor to help determine whether you're working too hard or not hard enough, what training zone or effort level you are working in, whether your recovery is complete, and how your fitness is progressing.

As with most of the other measures of intensity, heart-rate training zones are best used when tied to the standard of lactate threshold (LT). Often maximum heart rate is used as an estimate of LT, but that presents some problems. Attempting to achieve the highest heart rate possible in a workout requires extremely high motivation. In addition, for some individuals, exercising at such intensity may not be safe. Your true LT is a better indicator of what the body is experiencing and is highly variable from one athlete to the next. For example, your lactate-threshold heart rate (LTHR) may occur at 85 percent of maximum heart rate while another athlete's may be found at 92 percent. If both of you train at 90 percent of maximum, one is deeply anaerobic and working quite hard, but the other is cruising along, primarily in aerobic zones. Using the percentage of maximum heart rate to define your workout goal just isn't as precise as using zones based on LTHR. Finding your LTHR requires some effort, but don't let that scare you away. It's actually a simple procedure and is described in Appendix B under "Lactate-Threshold Test".

Just as with LT, heart rate zones vary by sport, since there are differences in the amount of muscle used and the effects of gravity among the different sports. For most triathletes, for example, LTHR is highest for running and lowest for swimming, with cycling in between. Lactate production also varies with the activity. This means that each sport must have its own set of heart rate values.

Power

Put simply, power is the ability to apply muscular strength. More precisely, it can be defined as Power = force × distance ÷ time. On the bike, if you are able to increase the gear size while your cadence remains constant, your power goes up. Your power also increases if you are able to turn the cranks faster with the same gear size. Currently it's not feasible to directly measure power in most other sports, although the day is rapidly approaching for running and may soon come to swimming, Nordic skiing, and others. For cycling, however, a power meter is a worthwhile investment, because power is more closely related to performance than any other measure discussed here, and it is therefore an excellent indicator of training workload.

The more power you can generate aerobically, the more likely you are to get good results in races. For example, according to one study, the amount of power generated during a 2-minute test is a better indicator of time trial ability on the bike than aerobic capacity (VO_2max). With a power meter, an athlete can compare heart rate to watts. Instead of just relying on how he or she feels, the athlete has objective information for establishing intensity.

Power meters remove most of the guesswork that goes into training and racing. For example, many athletes don't consider a work interval to be started until their heart rate reaches the targeted level. With a power meter, the interval starts as soon as the power hits the targeted zone—which means right away.

Heart rate monitors teach athletes to focus on the heart, but the muscles are really the key to fitness. This is particularly true when doing intervals. It can be very challenging to get the intensity right in the first minute or so of the first few intervals in a workout. Heart rate can't be relied upon because it lags behind; at the start of an interval it is low and takes a couple of minutes to rise. But a power meter identifies your intensity level precisely and immediately.

Using a power meter in a long race is almost like cheating. When everyone else is fighting the wind, or flying downwind, or guessing how hard to go when climbing, the athlete with a power meter is just rolling along at the prescribed power. He or she will produce the fastest possible effort because the optimal target power has been determined through training and then followed closely during the race. While something similar can be done with heart rate, there are some confounding factors, such as cardiac drift, the acute effect of diet, and the heart's slow response on hills.

Power meters also provide a highly accurate profile of how fitness changes throughout the season. When I was coaching athletes, I tested them regularly using a combination of heart rate and power. Without this information I really would not have known for sure whether they were making progress. I would have just been guessing.

Training with power, just as training with pace, RPE, or a heart rate monitor, requires the use of training zones based on a personal standard.

Lactate

If lactate threshold is such an important phenomenon, why not simply measure blood lactate to gauge intensity? Until recently, it wasn't practical to check lactate levels in the real world of endurance athletes. The only equipment available was expensive, cumbersome, and best suited for lab use. Today, there are lactate-measuring devices and mail-in services available, making it possible to measure lactate from a drop of blood drawn from the finger or earlobe. Such testing is still rather sophisticated and is reliable only in the hands of an experienced technician or coach. I would not recommend it for the self-coached athlete.

Lactate measurement does not provide instantaneous feedback in the same way that power, pace, and RPE do, since it takes a minute or two, at best, to draw and analyze the blood. At a couple of dollars per analysis, frequent measurement, even with a portable analyzer, is impractical. So lactate measurement is best used in a testing situation. It can be used to confirm LT, measure improvement, determine economy of movement, or set up a bike for optimal efficiency, for example.

Notes

Chapter 1: The Aging Myth

1. H. Kaplan, K. Hill, J. Lancaster, and A. M. Hurtado, "A Theory of Human Life History Evolution: Diet, Intelligence and Longevity," *Evolutionary Anthropology* 9 (4) (2000): 156–185.

2. L. B. Ransdell, J. Vener, and J. Huberty, "Masters Athletes: An Analysis of Running, Swimming and Cycling Performance by Age and Gender," *Journal of Exercise Science and Fitness* 7 (2) (2009): S61–S73.

3. R. Cox, "Record Breakers: 2013 Kona Age Group Records," Coach Cox, October 21, 2013, www.coachcox.co.uk/2013/10/21/record-breakers-2013-kona-age-group-records.

4. V. Y. Wright and B. C. Perricelli, "Age-Related Rates of Decline in Performance Among Elite Senior Athletes," *American Journal of Sports Medicine* 36 (3) (2008): 443–450.

5. H. Tanaka and D. R. Seals, "Age and Gender Interactions in Physiological Functional Capacity: Insight from Swimming Performance," *Journal of Applied Physiology* 82 (3) (1997): 846–851.

6. A. J. Donato, K. Tench, D. H. Glueck, D. R. Seals, I. Eskurza, and H. Tanaka, "Declines in Physiological Functional Capacity with Age: A Longitudinal Study in Peak Swimming Performance," *Journal of Applied Physiology* 94 (2) (2003): 764–769; J. T. Fairbrother, "Prediction of 1500-m Freestyle Swimming Times for Older Masters All-American Swimmers," *Experimental Aging Research* 33 (4) (2007): 461–471.

7. R. Lepers, F. Sultana, T. Bernard, C. Hausswirth, and J. Brisswalter, "Age-Related Changes in Triathlon Performances," *International Journal of Sports Medicine* 31 (4) (2010): 251–256.

8. M. L. Pollock, H. S. Miller, A. C. Linnerud, and K. H. Cooper, "Frequency of Training as a Determinant for Improvement in Cardiovascular Function and Body Composition of Middle-Aged Men," *Archives of Physical Medicine and Rehabilitation* 56 (4) (1975): 141–145.

9. T. Meyer, M. Auracher, K. Heeg, A. Urhausen, and W. Kindermann, "Effectiveness of Low-Intensity Endurance Training," *International Journal of Sports Medicine* 28 (1) (2007): 33–39; S. Seiler and E. Tonnessen, "Intervals, Thresholds, and Long Slow Distance: The Role of Intensity and Duration in Endurance Training," *Sportscience* 13 (2009): 32–53.

10. D. B. Dill, S. Robinson, and J. C. Ross, "A Longitudinal Study of 16 Champion Runners," *Journal of Sports Medicine and Physical Fitness* 7 (1) (1967): 4–27.

11. D. Lash, *The Iron Man from Indiana: The Don Lash Story* (Paducah, KY: Turner Publishing Co., 1999).

12. M. L. Pollock, C. Foster, D. Knapp, J. L. Rod, and D. H. Schmidt, "Effect of Age and Training on Aerobic Capacity and Body Composition of Masters Athletes," *Journal of Applied Physiology* 62 (2) (1987): 727–728.

13. M. L. Pollock, L. J. Mengelkoch, J. E. Graves, D. T. Lowenthal, M. C. Limacher, C. Foster, and J. H. Wilmore, "Twenty-Year Follow-up of Aerobic Power and Body Composition of Older Track Athletes," *Journal of Applied Physiology* 82 (5) (1997): 1508–1516.

14. M. A. Rogers, J. M. Hagberg, W. H. Martin III, A. A. Ehsani, and J. O. Holloszy, "Decline in VO₂max with Aging in Master Athletes and Sedentary Men," *Journal of Applied Physiology* 68 (5) (1990): 2195–2199; S. W. Trappe, D. L. Costill, M. D. Vukovich, J. Jones, and T. Melham, "Aging Among Elite Distance Runners: A 22-Yr Longitudinal Study," *Journal of Applied Physiology* 80 (1) (1996): 285–290; B. Marti and H. Howald, "Long-Term Effects of Physical Training on Aerobic Capacity: Controlled Study of Former Elite Athletes," *Journal of Applied Physiology* 69 (4) (1990): 1451–1459; L. I. Katzel, J. D. Sorkin, and J. L. Fleg, "A Comparison of Longitudinal Changes in Aerobic Fitness in Older Endurance Athletes and Sedentary Men," *Journal of the American Geriatric Society* 49 (12) (2001): 1657–1664.

15. Katzel, Sorkin, and Fleg, "A Comparison of Longitudinal Changes."

16. A. E. Pimentel, C. L. Gentile, H. Tanaka, D. R. Seals, and P. E. Gates, "Greater Rate of Decline in Maximal Aerobic Capacity with Age in Endurance-Trained Than in Sedentary Men," *Journal of Applied Physiology* 94 (6) (2003): 2406–2413.

17. D. R. Seals, B. F. Hurley, J. Schultz, and J. M. Hagberg, "Endurance Training in Older Men and Women II: Blood Lactate Response to Submaximal Exercise," *Journal of Applied Physiology* 57 (4) (1984): 1030–1033.

18. H. A. De Vries, "Physiological Effects of an Exercise Training Regimen upon Men Aged 52 to 88," *Journal of Gerontology* 25 (4) (1970): 325–336; J. Orlander and A. Aniansson, "Effect of Physical Training on Skeletal Muscle Metabolism and Ultrastructure in 70 to 75-Year-Old Men," *Acta Physiolica Scandinavica* 109 (2) (1980): 149–154.

Chapter 2: The Ageless Athlete

1. C. Rosenbloom and M. Bahns, "What Can We Learn About Diet and Physical Activity from Master Athletes?" *Holistic Nursing Practice* 20 (4) (2006): 161–166.

2. Ibid.

3. P. Reaburn and B. Dascombe, "Endurance Performance in Masters Athletes," *European Review of Aging and Physical Activity* 5 (2008): 31–42; R. A. Dionigi, J. Baker, and S. Horton, "Older Athletes' Perceived Benefits of Competition," *International Journal of Sport and Society* 2 (2) (2010): 17–28.

4. I. M. Lee and P. J. Skerrett, "Physical Activity and All-Cause Mortality: What Is the Dose-Response Relation?" *Medicine and Science in Sports and Exercise* 33 (6S) (2001): S459–471.

5. Ibid.; R. S. Paffenbarger, Jr., R. T. Hyde, A. L. Wing, and C. C. Hsieh, "Physical Activity, All-Cause Mortality, and Longevity of College Alumni," *New England Journal of Medicine* 314 (10) (1986): 605–613.

6. Lee and Skerrett, "Physical Activity and All-Cause Mortality."

7. Stefan Mohlenkamp, Nils Lehmann, Frank Breuckmann, Martina Bröcker-Preuss, Kai Nassenstein, Martin Halle, Thomas Budde, Klaus Mann, Jörg Barkhausen, Gerd Heusch, Karl-Heinz Jöckel, and Raimund Erbe, "Running: The Risk of Coronary Events—Prevalence and Prognostic Relevance of Coronary Atherosclerosis in Marathon Runners," *European Heart Journal* 29 (2008): 1903–1910; J. H. O'Keefe, H. R. Patil, C. J. Lavie, A. Magalski, R. A. Vogel, and P. A. McCullough, "Potential Adverse Cardiovascular Effects from Excessive Endurance Exercise," *Mayo Clinic Proceedings* 87 (6) (2012): 587–595; P. Schnohr, J. L. Marott, P. Lange, and G. B. Jensen, "Longevity in Male and Female Joggers: The Copenhagen City Heart Study," *American Journal of Epidemiology* 177 (7) (2013): 683–689.

8. T. Noakes, "Time to Quit That Marathon Running? Not Quite Yet!" *Basic Research in Cardiology* 109 (2014): 395–396.

9. A. Safdar, J. Bourgeois, D. I. Ogburn, J. P. Little, B. P. Hettinga, M. Akhtar, J. E. Thompson, S. Melov, N. J. Mocellin, G. C. Kujoth, T. A. Prolla, and M. A. Tarnopolsky, "Endurance Exercise Rescues Progeroid Aging and Induces Systemic Mitochondrial Rejuvenation in mtDNA Mutator Mice," *Proceedings of the National Academy of Sciences USA* 108 (10) (2011): 4135–4140.

10. T. J. LaRocca, D. R. Seals, and G. L. Pierce, 'Leukocyte Telomere Length Is Preserved with Aging in Endurance Exercise-Trained Adults and Related to Maximal Aerobic Capacity," *Mechanisms of Ageing and Development* 131 (2) (2010): 165–167.

11. A. T. Ludlow and S. M. Roth, "Physical Activity and Telomere Biology: Exploring the Link with Aging-Related Disease Prevention," *Journal of Aging Research* (2011): 790378.

12. T. C. J. Tan, R. Rahman, F. Jaber-Hijazi, D. A. Felix, C. Chen, E. J. Louis, and A. Aboobaker, "Telomere Maintenance and Telomerase Activity Are Differentially Regulated in Asexual and Sexual Worms," *Proceedings of the National Academy of Sciences USA* 109 (11) (2012): 4209–4214.

13. B. Balk, A. Maicher, M. Dees, J. Klermund, S. Luke-Glaser, K. Bender, and B. Luke, "Telomeric RNA-DNA Hybrids Affect Telomere-Length Dynamics and Senescence," *Nature Structural and Molecular Biology* 20 (10) (2013): 1199–1205.

14. D. Hanahan and R. A. Weinberg, "The Hallmarks of Cancer," *Cell* 100 (1) (2000): 57–70.

15. L. C. Chosewood, "Safer and Healthier at Any Age: Strategies for an Aging Workforce," *NIOSH Science Blog*, July 19, 2012, National Institute for Occupational Safety and Health, http://blogs.cdc.gov/niosh-science-blog/2012/07/19/agingworkforce/.

16. John R. Speakman, "Body Size, Energy Metabolism and Lifespan," *Journal of Experimental Biology* 208 (9) (2005): 1717–1730.

17. D. Gems and L. Partridge, "Genetics of Longevity in Model Organisms: Debates and Paradigm Shifts," *Annual Review of Physiology* 75 (2013): 621–644.

18. J. M. Gutteridge and B. Halliwell, "Free Radicals and Antioxidants in the Year 2000: A Historical Look to the Future," *Annals of the New York Academy of Sciences* 899 (2000): 136–147.

19. V. I. Pérez, A. Bokov, H. V. Remmen, J. Mele, Q. Ran, Y. Ikeno, and A. Richardson, "Is the Oxidative Stress Theory of Aging Dead?" *Biochimica et Biophysica Acta* 1790 (10) (2009): 1005–1014.

20. Gems and Partridge, "Genetics of Longevity in Model Organisms";. P. Jha, M. Flather, E. Lonn, M. Farkouh, and S. Yusuf, "The Antioxidant Vitamins and Cardiovascular Disease: A Critical Review of Epidemiologic and Clinical Trial Data,"*Annals of Internal Medicine* 123 (11) (1995): 860–872; G. Bjelakovic, D. Nikolova, L. L. Gluud, R. G. Simonetti, and C. Gluud, "Mortality in Randomized Trials of Antioxidant Supplements for Primary and Secondary Prevention: Systematic Review and Meta-analysis," *Journal of the American Medical Association* 297 (8) (2007): 842–857.

21. M. M. Vilenchik and A. G. Knudson, Jr., "Inverse Radiation Dose-Rate Effects on Somatic and Germ-Line Mutations and DNA Damage Rates," *Proceedings of the National Acadamy of Sciences USA* 97 (2000): 5381–5386.

22. B. P. Best, "Nuclear DNA Damage as a Direct Cause of Aging," *Rejuvenation Research* 12 (3) (2009): 199–208.

23. World Health Organization, "WHO Life Expectancy: Life Expectancy by Country," 2013, http://apps.who.int/gho/data/node.main.688?lang=en.

24. D. Baker, T. Wijshake, T. Tchkonia, N. K. LeBrasseur, B. G. Childs, B. van de Sluis, J. L. Kirkland, and J. M. van Deursen, "Clearance of p16Ink4a-Positive Senescent Cells Delays Ageing-Associated Disorders," *Nature* 479 (7372) (2011): 232–236.

25. G. Shefer, G. Rauner, Z. Yablonka-Reuveni, and D. Benayahu, "Reduced Satellite Cell Numbers and Myogenic Capacity in Aging Can Be Alleviated by Endurance Exercise," *PLoS One* 5 (10) (2010): e13307.

26. F. Kadi, N. Charifi, C. Denis, J. Lexell, J. L. Andersen, P. Schjerling, S. Olsen, and M. Kjaer, "The Behaviour of Satellite Cells in Response to Exercise: What Have We Learned from Human Studies?" *Pflügers Archiv—European Journal of Physiology* 451 (2005): 319–327; R. Crameri, P. Aagaard, K. Qvortrup, and M. Kjaer, "N-CAM and Pax7 Immunoreactive Cells Are Expressed Differently in the Human Vastus Lateralis After a Single Bout of Exhaustive Eccentric Exercise," *Journal of Physiology* 565 (2004): 165.

27. M. M. Bamman, J. R. Shipp, J. Jiang, B. A. Gower, G. R. Hunter, A. Goodman, C. L. McLafferty, Jr., and R. J. Urban, "Mechanical Load Increases Muscle IGF-I and Androgen Receptor mRNA Concentrations in Humans," *American Journal of Physiology* 280 (2001): 383–390; Y. Hellsten, H. A. Hansson, L. Johnson, U. Frandsen, and B. Sjödin, "Increased Expression of Xanthine Oxidase and Insulin-Like Growth Factor I (IGF-I) Immunoreactivity in Skeletal Muscle After Strenuous Exercise in Humans," *Acta Physiologica Scandinavica* 157 (1996): 191–197.

28. N. Charifi, F. Kadi, L. Feasson, and C. Denis, "Effects of Endurance Training on Satellite Cell Frequency in Skeletal Muscle of Old Men," *Muscle Nerve* 28 (2003): 87–92.

29. D. C. Willcox, B. J. Willcox, W. C. Hsueh, and M. Suzuki, "Genetic Determinants of Exceptional Human Longevity: Insights from the Okinawa Centenarian Study," *Age* 28 (4) (2006): 313–332.

30. H. Shibata, H. Nagai, H. Haga, S. Yasumura, T. Suzuki, and Y. Suyama, "Nutrition for the Japanese Elderly," *Nutrition and Health* 8 (2–3) (1992): 165–175.

31. B. J. Willcox, D. C. Willcox, H. Todoriki, A. Fujiyoshi, K. Yano, Q. He, J. D. Curb, and M. Suzuki, "Caloric Restriction, the Traditional Okinawan Diet, and Healthy Aging: The Diet of the World's Longest-Lived People and Its Potential Impact on Morbidity and Life Span," *Annals of the New York Academy of Sciences* 1114 (2007): 434–455.

32. D. F. Lawler, B. T. Larson, J. M. Ballam, G. K. Smith, D. N. Biery, R. H. Evans, E. H. Greeley, M. Segre, H. D. Stowe, and R. D. Kealy, "Diet Restriction and Ageing in the Dog: Major Observations over Two Decades," *British Journal of Nutrition* 99 (4) (2008): 793–805; A. V. Everitt and D. G. Le Couteur, "Life Extension by Calorie Restriction in Humans," *Annals of the New York Academy of Sciences* 1114 (2007): 428–433.

33. N. Onishi, "Love of U.S. Food Shortening Okinawans' Lives: Life Expectancy Among Island's Young Men Takes a Big Dive," *San Francisco Chronicle*, April 4, 2004, http://www.sfgate.com/health/article/Love-of-U-S-food-shortening-Okinawans-lives-2397590.php#page-1.

34. Ibid.; Y. Kagawa, "Impact of Westernization on the Nutrition of Japanese: Changes in Physique, Cancer, Longevity and Centenarians," *Preventive Medicine* 7 (2) (1978): 205–217.

Chapter 3: Over the Hill

1. S. K. Hunter, A. A. Stevens, K. Magennis, K. W. Skelton, and M. Fauth, "Is There a Sex Difference in the Age of Elite Marathon Runners?" *Medicine and Science in Sports and Exercise* 43 (4) (2011): 656–664.

2. B. W. Young and J. L. Starkes, "Career-Span Analyses of Track Performance: Longitudinal Data Present a More Optimistic View of Age-Related Performance Decline," *Experimental Aging Research* 31 (1) (2005): 69–90; B. W. Young, P. L. Weir, J. L. Starkes, and N. Medic, "Does Lifelong Training Temper Age-Related Decline in Sport Performance? Interpreting Differences Between Cross-Sectional and Longitudinal Data," *Experimental Aging Research* 34 (1) (2008): 27–48; C. Heavens, "Dr. Vonda Wright: From Orthopedic Surgeon to Fitness Expert, Dr. Vonda Wright Keeps Fitness on Track for the over-40 Crowd," *Pittsburgh Magazine*, September 14, 2010, http: //www.pittsburghmagazine.com/Pittsburgh-Magazine/March-2009/Dr-Vonda-Wright/; V. J. Wright, "Masterful Care of the Aging Triathlete," *Sports Medicine and Arthroscopy Review* 20 (4) (2012): 231–236.

3. L. V. Billat and J. P. Koralsztein, "Significance of the Velocity at VO_2max and Time to Exhaustion at this Velocity," *Sports Medicine* 22 (2) (1996): 90–108; V. Billat, M. Faina, F. Sardella, C. Marini, F. Fanton, S. Lupo, P. Faccini, M. de Angelis, J. P. Koralsztein, and A. Dalmonte, "A Comparison of Time to Exhaustion at VO_2 max in Élite Cyclists, Kayak Paddlers, Swimmers and Runners," *Ergonomics* 39 (2) (1996): 267–277; R. J. Fernandes, K. L. Keskinen, P. Colaço, A. J. Querido, L. J. Machado, P. A. Morais, D. Q. Novais, D. A. Marinho, and J. P. Vilas-Boas, "Time Limit at VO_2max Velocity in Elite Crawl Swimmers," *International Journal of Sports Medicine* 29 (2) (2008): 145–150.

4. N. Uth, H. Sørensen, K. Overgaard, and P. K. Pedersen, "Estimation of VO_2max from the Ratio Between HRmax and HRrest—the Heart Rate Ratio Method," *European Journal of Applied Physiology* 91 (1) (2004): 111–115.

5. C. Bouchard, R. Lesage, G. Lortie, J. A. Simoneau, P. Hamel, M. R. Boulay, L. Perusse, G. Theriault, and C. Leblanc, "Aerobic Performance in Brothers, Dizygotic and Monozygotic Twins," *Medicine and Science in Sports and Exercise* 18 (6) (1986): 639–646.

6. B. M. Nes, I. Janszky, L. J. Vatten, T. I. Nilsen, S. T. Aspenes, and U. Wisløff, "Estimating VO_2 Peak from a Nonexercise Prediction Model: The HUNT Study, Norway," *Medicine and Science in Sports and Exercise* 43 (11) 2011: 2024–2030.

7. L. G. Koch, O. J. Kemi, N. Qi, S. X. Leng, P. Bijma, L. J. Gilligan, J. E. Wilkinson, H. Wisloff, M. A. Hoydal, N. Rolim, P. M. Abadir, E. M. Van Grevenhof, G. L. Smith, C. F. Burant, O. Ellingsen, S. L. Britton, and U. Wisloff, "Intrinsic Aerobic Capacity Sets a Divide for Aging and Longevity," *Circulation Research* 109 (10) (2011): 1162–1172.

8. K. Wasserman and A. Koike, "Is the Anaerobic Threshold Truly Anaerobic?" *Chest* 101 (5 Suppl.) (1992): 211S–218S.

9. E. F. Coyle, "Integration of the Physiological Factors Determining Endurance Performance Ability," *Exercise and Sport Sciences Reviews* 23 (1995): 25–63.

10. Hunter Allen and Andrew Coggan, *Training and Racing with a Power Meter*, 2nd ed. (Boulder, CO: VeloPress, 2010).

11. T. Noakes, *The Lore of Running*, 4th ed. (Champaign, IL: Human Kinetics, 2003).

12. K. R. Williams, "Biomechanical Factors Contributing to Marathon Race Success," *Sports Medicine* 37 (4–5) (2007): 420–423.

13. Noakes, *The Lore of Running*.

14. Ibid.

15. Ibid.; Williams, "Biomechanical Factors Contributing to Marathon Race Success"; E. C. Frederick, "Physiological and Ergonomics Factors in Running Shoe Design," *Applied Ergonomics* 15 (4) (1984): 281–287.

16. G. Jagomägi and T. Jürimäe, "The Influence of Anthropometrical and Flexibility Parameters on the Results of Breaststroke Swimming," *Anthropologischer Anzeiger* 63 (2) (2005): 213–219.

17. G. R. Hunter, K. Katsoulis, J. P. McCarthy, W. K. Ogard, M. M. Bamman, D. S. Wood, J. A. Den Hollander, T. E. Blaudeau, and B. R. Newcomer, "Tendon Length and Joint Flexibility Are Related to Running Economy," *Medicine and Science in Sports and Exercise* 43 (8) (2011): 1492–1499.

18. J. Franch, K. Madsen, M. S. Djurhuus, and P. K. Pedersen, "Improved Running Economy Following Intensified Training Correlates with Reduced Ventilatory Demands," *Medicine and Science in Sports and Exercise* 30 (8) (1998): 1250–1256; J. Slawinski, A. Demarle, J. P. Koralsztein, and V. Billat, "Effect of Supra-lactate Threshold Training on the Relationship Between Mechanical Stride Descriptors and Aerobic Energy Cost in Trained Runners," *Archives of Physiology and Biochemistry* 109 (2) (2001): 110–116.

19. R. W. Spurrs, A. J. Murphy, and M. L. Watsford, "The Effect of Plyometric Training on Distance Running Performance," *European Journal of Applied Physiology* 89 (1) (2003): 1–7; P. U. Saunders, R. D. Telford, D. B. Pyne, E. M. Peltola, R. B. Cunningham, C. J. Gore, and J. A. Hawley, "Short-Term Plyometric Training Improves Running Economy in Highly Trained Middle and Long Distance Runners," *Journal of Strength and Conditioning Research* 20 (4) (2006): 947–954; A. M. Turner, M. Owings, and J. A. Schwane, "Improvement in Running Economy After 6 Weeks of Plyometric Training," *Journal of Strength and Conditioning Research* 17 (1) (2003): 60–67; C. D. Paton and W. G. Hopkins, "Combining Explosive and High-Resistance Training Improves Performance in Competitive Cyclists," *Journal of Strength and Conditioning Research* 19 (4) (2005): 826–830.

20. A. P. Jung, "The Impact of Resistance Training on Distance Running Performance," *Sports Medicine* 33 (7) (2003): 539–552; J. Hoff, J. Helgerud, and U. Wisløff, "Maximal Strength Training Improves Work Economy in Trained Female Cross-Country Skiers," *Medicine and Science in Sports and Exercise* 31 (6) (1999): 870–877; D. J. Loveless, C. L. Weber, L. J. Haseler, and D. A. Schneider, "Maximal Leg-Strength Training Improves Cycling Economy in Previously Untrained Men," *Medicine and Science in Sports and Exercise* 37 (7) (2005): 1231–1236.

21. D. Bishop, D. G. Jenkins, L. T. Mackinnon, M. McEniery, and M. F. Carey, "The Effects of Strength Training on Endurance Performance and Muscle Characteristics," *Medicine and Science in Sports and Exercise* 31 (6) (1999): 886–891; N. P. Jackson, M. S. Hickey, and R. F. Reiser II, "High Resistance/Low Repetition vs. Low Resistance/High Repetition Training: Effects on Performance of Trained Cyclists," *Journal of Strength and Conditioning Research* 21 (1) (2007): 289–295; A. Ferrauti, M. Bergermann, and J. Fernandez-Fernandez, "Effects of a Concurrent Strength and Endurance Training on Running Performance and Running Economy in Recreational Marathon Runners," *Journal of Strength and Conditioning Research* 24 (10) (2010): 2770–2778.

22. A. Lucía, J. Hoyos, M. Pérez, A. Santalla, and J. L. Chicharro, "Inverse Relationship Between VO_2max and Economy/Efficiency in World-Class Cyclists," *Medicine and Science in Sports and Exercise* 34 (12) (2002): 2079–2084; D. L. Conley and G. S. Krahenbuhl, "Running Economy and Distance Running Performance of Highly Trained Athletes," *Medicine and Science in Sports and Exercise* 12 (5) (1980): 357–360; P. U. Saunders, D. B. Pyne, R. D. Telford, and J. A. Hawley, "Factors Affecting Running Economy in Trained Distance Runners," *Sports Medicine* 34 (7) (2004): 465–485.

23. H. Tanaka and D. R. Seals, "Invited Review: Dynamic Exercise Performance in Masters Athletes: Insight into the Effects of Primary Human Aging on Physiological Functional Capacity," *Journal of Applied Physiology* 95 (5) (2003): 2152–2162; H. Tanaka and D. R. Seals, "Endurance Exercise Performance in Masters Athletes: Age-Associated Changes and Underlying Physiological Mecha-

nisms," *Journal of Physiology* 586 (1) (2008): 55–63; R. A. Wiswell, V. Jaque, T. J. Marcell, S. A. Hawkins, K. M. Tarpenning, N. Constantino, and D. M. Hyslop, "Maximal Aerobic Power, Lactate Threshold, and Running Performance in Master Athletes," *Medicine and Science in Sports and Exercise* 32 (2000): 1165–1170.

24. T. J. Quinn, M. J. Manley, J. Aziz, J. M. Padham, and A. M. MacKenzie, "Aging and Factors Related to Running Economy," *Journal of Strength and Conditioning Research* 25 (11) (2011): 2971–2979.

25. Tanaka and Seals, "Invited Review: Dynamic Exercise Performance in Masters Athletes"; Tanaka and Seals, "Endurance Exercise Performance in Masters Athletes"; Wiswell et al., "Maximal Aerobic Power, Lactate Threshold, and Running Performance in Master Athletes."

26. M. L. Pollock, C. Foster, D. Knapp, J. L. Rod, and D. H. Schmidt, "Effect of Age and Training on Aerobic Capacity and Body Composition of Master Athletes," *Journal of Applied Physiology* 62 (2) (1987): 725–731.

27. Wiswell et al., "Maximal Aerobic Power, Lactate Threshold, and Running Performance in Master Athletes"; W. K. Allen, D. R. Seals, B. F. Hurley, A. A. Ehsani, and J. M. Hagberg, "Lactate Threshold and Distance-Running Performance in Young and Older Endurance Athletes," *Journal of Applied Physiology* 58 (4) (1985): 1281–1284.

28. D. R. Bassett, Jr., and E. T. Howley, "Limiting Factors for Maximum Oxygen Uptake and Determinants of Endurance Performance," *Medicine and Science in Sports and Exercise* 32 (1) (2000): 70–84.

29. P. D. Wagner, "New Ideas on Limitations to VO_2max," *Exercise and Sport Sciences Reviews* 28 (1) (2000): 10–14; T. M. Wilson and H. Tanaka, "Meta-analysis of the Age-Associated Decline in Maximal Aerobic Capacity in Men: Relation to Training Status," *American Journal of Physiology— Heart and Circulatory Physiology* 278 (3) (2000): H829–834.

30. S. Pfaffenberger, P. Bartko, A. Graf, E. Pernicka, J. Babayev, E. Lolic, D. Bonderman, H. Baumgartner, G. Maurer, and J. Mascherbauer, "Size Matters! Impact of Age, Sex, Height, and Weight on the Normal Heart Size," *Circulation: Cardiovascular Imaging* 6 (6) (2013): 1073–1079; D. R. Seals, J. M. Hagberg, R. J. Spina, M. A. Rogers, K. B. Schechtman, and A. A. Ehsani, "Enhanced Left Ventricular Performance in Endurance Trained Older Men," *Circulation* 89 (1) (1994): 198–205.

31. Billat et al., "Significance of the Velocity at VO_2max and Time to Exhaustion at this Velocity."

32. J. L. Fleg, C. H. Morrell, A. G. Bos, L. J. Brant, L. A. Talbot, J. G. Wright, and E. G. Lakatta, "Accelerated Longitudinal Decline of Aerobic Capacity in Healthy Older Adults," *Circulation* 112 (5) (2005): 674–682.

33. E. D. Larson, J. R. St. Clair, W. A. Sumner, R. A. Bannister, and C. Proenza, "Depressed Pacemaker Activity of Sinoatrial Node Myocytes Contributes to the Age-Dependent Decline in Maximum Heart Rate," *Proceedings of the National Academy of Sciences USA* 110 (44) (2013): 18011–18016; G. W. Heath, J. M. Hagberg, A. A. Ehsani, and J. O. Holloszy, "A Physiological Comparison of Young and Older Endurance Athletes," *Journal of Applied Physiology: Respiratory, Environmental, and Exercise Physiology* 51 (3) (1981): 634–640; S. A. Hawkins, T. J. Marcell, S. Victoria Jaque, and R. A. Wiswell, "A Longitudinal Assessment of Change in VO_2max and Maximal Heart Rate in Masters Athletes," *Medicine and Science in Sports and Exercise* 33 (10) (2001): 1744–1750.

34. Hawkins et al., "A Longitudinal Assessment of Change in VO_2max and Maximal Heart Rate in Masters Athletes"; C. L. Wells, M.A. Boorman, and D. M. Riggs, "Effect of Age and Menopausal Status on Cardiorespiratory Fitness in Masters Women Runners," *Medicine and Science in Sports and Exercise* 24 (10) (1992): 1147–1154.

35. M. A. Rogers, J. M. Hagberg, W. H. Martin III, A. A. Ehsani, and J. O. Holloszy, "Decline in VO₂max with Aging in Master Athletes and Sedentary Men," *Journal of Applied Physiology* 68 (5) (1990): 2195–2199.

36. Wagner, "New Ideas on Limitations to VO₂max."

37. S. Hawkins and R. Wiswell, "Rate and Mechanism of Maximal Oxygen Consumption Decline with Aging: Implications for Exercise Training," *Sports Medicine* 33 (12) (2003): 877–888.

38. M. F. Rolland-Cachera, T. J. Cole, M. Sempé, J. Tichet, C. Rossignol, and A. Charraud, "Body Mass Index Variations: Centiles from Birth to 87 Years," *European Journal of Clinical Nutrition* 45 (1) (1991): 13–21.

39. G. B. Forbes and J. C. Reina, "Adult Lean Body Mass Declines with Age: Some Longitudinal Observations," *Metabolism* 19 (9) (1970): 653–663.

40. K. R. Short, J. L. Vittone, M. L. Bigelow, D. N. Proctor, and K. S. Nair, "Age and Aerobic Exercise Training Effects on Whole Body and Muscle Protein Metabolism," *American Journal of Physiology—Endocrinology and Metabolism* 286 (1) (2004): E92-E101.

41. F. F. Horber, S. A. Kohler, K. Lippuner, and P. Jaeger, "Effect of Regular Physical Training on Age-Associated Alteration of Body Composition in Men," *European Journal of Clinical Investigation* 26 (4) (1996): 279–285.

42. L. D. Ferreira, L. K. Pulawa, D. R. Jensen, and R. H. Eckel, "Overexpressing Human Lipoprotein Lipase in Mouse Skeletal Muscle Is Associated with Insulin Resistance," *Diabetes* 50 (5) (2001): 1064–1068; J. K. Kim, J. J. Fillmore, Y. Chen, C. Yu, I. K. Moore, M. Pypaert, E. P. Lutz, Y. Kako, W. Velez-Carrasco, I. J. Goldberg, J. I. Breslow, and G. I. Shulman, "Tissue-Specific Overexpression of Lipoprotein Lipase Causes Tissue-Specific Insulin Resistance," *Proceedings of the National Academy of Sciences USA* 98 (13) (2001): 7522–7527; J. Delezie, S. Dumont, H. Dardente, H. Oudart, A. Gréchez-Cassiau, P. Klosen, M. Teboul, F. Delaunay, P. Pévet, and E. Challet, "The Nuclear Receptor REV-ERB™ Is Required for the Daily Balance of Carbohydrate and Lipid Metabolism," *FASEB Journal* 26 (8) (2012): 3321–3335; A. Ferland, M. L. Château-Degat, T. L. Hernandez, and R. H. Eckel, "Tissue-Specific Responses of Lipoprotein Lipase to Dietary Macronutrient Composition as a Predictor of Weight Gain over 4 Years," *Obesity* 20 (5) (2012): 1006–1011.

43. T. J. Yost, D. R. Jensen, and R. H. Eckel, "Tissue-Specific Lipoprotein Lipase: Relationships to Body Composition and Body Fat Distribution in Normal Weight Humans," *Obesity Research* 1 (1) (1993): 1–4.

44. I. Janssen, S. B. Heymsfield, Z. Wang, and R. Ross, "Skeletal Muscle Mass and Distribution in 468 Men and Women Aged 18–88 Yr.," *Journal of Applied Physiology* 89 (2000): 81–88; J. G. Ryall, J. D. Schertzer, and G. S. Lynch, "Cellular and Molecular Mechanisms Underlying Age-Related Skeletal Muscle Wasting and Weakness," *Biogerontology* 9 (4) (2008): 213–228; T. N. Kim and K. M. Choi, "Sarcopenia: Definition, Epidemiology, and Pathophysiology," *Journal of Bone Metabolism* 20 (1) (2013): 1–10.

45. T. J. Doherty, "Invited Review: Aging and Sarcopenia," *Journal of Applied Physiology* 95 (4) (2003): 1717–1727; H. Karakelides and K. S. Nair, "Sarcopenia of Aging and Its Metabolic Impact," *Current Topics in Developmental Biology* 68 (2005): 123–148.

46. D. L. Waters, C. L. Yau, G. D. Montoya, and R. N. Baumgartner, "Serum Sex Hormones, IGF-1, and IGFBP3 Exert a Sexually Dimorphic Effect on Lean Body Mass in Aging," *Journals of Gerontology, Series A: Biological Sciences and Medical Sciences* 58 (7) (2003): 648–652.

47. V. Messier, R. Rabasa-Lhoret, S. Barbat-Artigas, B. Elisha, A. D. Karelis, and M. Aubertin-Leheudre, "Menopause and Sarcopenia: A Potential Role for Sex Hormones," *Maturitas* 68 (4) (2011): 331–336.

48. G. A. Power, B. H. Dalton, D. G. Behm, A. A. Vandervoort, T. J. Doherty, and C. L. Rice, "Motor Unit Number Estimates in Masters Runners: Use It or Lose It?" *Medicine and Science in Sports and Exercise* 42 (9) (2010): 1644–1650.

49. G. A. Power, B. H. Dalton, D. G. Behm, T. J. Doherty, A. A. Vandervoort, and C. L. Rice, "Motor Unit Number Survival in Lifelong Runners Is Muscle Dependent," *Medicine and Science in Sports and Exercise* 44 (7) (2012): 1235–1242.

50. A. Chalé, G. J. Cloutier, C. Hau, E. M. Phillips, G. E. Dallal, and R. A. Fielding, "Efficacy of Whey Protein Supplementation on Resistance Exercise-Induced Changes in Lean Mass, Muscle Strength, and Physical Function in Mobility-Limited Older Adults," *Journals of Gerontology, Series A: Biological Sciences and Medical Sciences* 68 (6) (2012): 682–690.

51. A. P. Wroblewski, F. Amati, M. A. Smiley, B. Goodpaster, and V. Wright, "Chronic Exercise Preserves Lean Muscle Mass in Masters Athletes," *Physician and Sports Medicine* 39 (30) (2011): 172–178; V. J. Wright, "Masterful Care of the Aging Triathlete," *Sports Medicine and Arthroscopy* 20 (4) (2012): 23–26.

52. J. A. Faulkner, C. S. Davis, C. L. Mendias, and S. V. Brooks, "The Aging of Elite Male Athletes: Age-Related Changes in Performance and Skeletal Muscle Structure and Function," *Clinical Journal of Sport Medicine* 18 (6) (2008): 501–507.

Chapter 4: The High-Performance Senior Athlete

1. D. Leyk, O. Erley, W. Gorges, D. Ridder, T. Rüther, M. Wunderlich, A. Sievert, D. Essfeld, C. Piekarski, and T. Erren, "Performance, Training and Lifestyle Parameters of Marathon Runners Aged 20–80 Years: Results of the PACE-Study," *International Journal of Sports Medicine* 30 (5) (2009): 360–365.

2. M. Lehman, H. Mann, U. Gastmann, J. Keul, D. Vetter, J. M. Steinacker, and D. Häussinger, "Unaccustomed High-Mileage vs Intensity Training-Related Changes in Performance and Serum Acid Levels," *International Journal of Sports Medicine* 17 (3) (1996): 187–192; P. B. Laursen and D. G. Jenkins, "The Scientific Basis for High-Intensity Interval Training: Optimizing Training Programmes and Maximizing Performance in Highly Trained Endurance Athletes," *Sports Medicine* 32 (1) (2002): 52–73; A. W. Midgley, L. R. McNaughton, and M. Wilkinson, "Is There an Optimal Training Intensity for Enhancing the Maximal Oxygen Uptake of Distance Runners? Empirical Research Findings, Current Opinions, Physiological Rationale and Practical Recommendations," *Sports Medicine* 36 (2) (2006): 117–132; J. Helgerud, K. Høydal, E. Wang, T. Karlsen, P. Berg, M. Bjerkaas, T. Simonsen, C. Helgesen, N. Hjorth, R. Bach, and J. Hoff, "Aerobic High-Intensity Intervals Improve VO$_2$max More Than Moderate Training," *Medicine and Science in Sports and Exercise* 39 (4) (2007): 665–671; I. Muñoz, S. Seiler, J. Bautista, J. España, E. Larumbe, and J. Esteve-Lanao, "Does Polarized Training Improve Performance in Recreational Runners?" *International Journal of Sports Physiology and Performance* 9 (2) (2013): 265–272.

3. R. Lepers, F. Sultana, T. Bernard, C. Hausswirth, and J. Brisswalter, "Age-Related Changes in Triathlon Performances," *International Journal of Sports Medicine* 31 (4) (2010): 251–256.

4. R. Lepers, "Gender and Age Considerations in Triathlon," in *Triathlon Science*, edited by J. Friel and J. Vance (Champaign, IL: Human Kinetics, 2013).

5. T. M. Wilson and H. Tanaka, "Meta-analysis of the Age-Associated Decline in Maximal Aerobic Capacity in Men: Relation to Training Status," *American Journal of Physiology—Heart and Circulatory Physiology* 278 (3) (2000): H829–834.

6. M. L. Pollock, C. Foster, D. Knapp, J. L. Rod, and D. H. Schmidt, "Effect of Age and Training on Aerobic Capacity and Body Composition of Masters Athletes," *Journal of Applied Physiology* 62 (2) (1987): 727–728.

7. E. Enoksen, S. A. Shalfawi, and E. Tønnessen, "The Effect of High- vs. Low-Intensity Training on Aerobic Capacity in Well-Trained Male Middle-Distance Runners," *Journal of Strength and Conditioning Research* 25 (3) (2011): 812–818.

8. F. Esfarjani and P. B. Laursen, "Manipulating High-Intensity Interval Training: Effects on VO$_2$max, the Lactate Threshold and 3000 m Running Performance in Moderately Trained Males," *Journal of Science and Medicine in Sport* 10 (1) (2007): 27–35; A. W. Midgley, L. R. McNaughton, and M. Wilkinson, "Is There an Optimal Training Intensity for Enhancing the Maximal Oxygen Uptake of Distance Runners? Empirical Research Findings, Current Opinions, Physiological Rationale and Practical Recommendations," *Sports Medicine* 36 (2) (2006): 117–132; A. W. Midgley and L. R. McNaughton, "Time at or Near VO$_2$max During Continuous and Intermittent Running: A Review with Special Reference to Considerations for the Optimisation of Training Protocols to Elicit the Longest Time at or Near VO$_2$max," *Journal of Sports Medicine and Physical Fitness* 46 (1) (2006): 1–14.

9. P. I. Brown, M. G. Hughes, and R. J. Tong, "The Effect of Warm-up on High-Intensity, Intermittent Running Using Nonmotorized Treadmill Ergometry," *Journal of Strength and Conditioning Research* 22 (3) (2008): 801–808.

10. L. J. Mengelkoch, M. L. Pollock, M. C. Limacher, J. E. Graves, R. B. Shireman, W. J. Riley, D. T. Lowenthal, and A. S. Leon, "Effects of Age, Physical Training, and Physical Fitness on Coronary Heart Disease Risk Factors in Older Track Athletes at Twenty-Year Follow-Up," *Journal of the American Geriatric Society* 45 (12) (1997): 1446–1453; O. Rognmo, T. Moholdt, H. Bakken, T. Hole, P. Mølstad, N. E. Myhr, J. Grimsmo, and U. Wisløff, "Cardiovascular Risk of High- Versus Moderate-Intensity Aerobic Exercise in Coronary Heart Disease Patients," *Circulation* 126 (12) (2012): 1436–1440.

11. L. V. Billat and J. P. Koralsztein, "Significance of the Velocity at VO$_2$max and Time to Exhaustion at this Velocity," *Sports Medicine* 22 (2) (1996): 90–108.

12. T. Eken and K. Gundersen, "Electrical Stimulation Resembling Normal Motor-Unit Activity: Effects on Denervated Fast and Slow Rat Muscles," *Journal of Physiology* 402 (1988): 651–669.

13. D. Pette and R. S. Staron, "Mammalian Skeletal Muscle Fiber Type Transitions," *International Review of Cytology* 170 (1997): 143–223.

14. V. I. Kalapotharakos, K. Diamantopoulos, and S. P. Tokmakidis, "Effects of Resistance Training and Detraining on Muscle Strength and Functional Performance of Older Adults Aged 80 to 88 Years," *Aging Clinical and Experimental Research* 22 (2) (2010): 134–140.

15. T. J. Quinn, M. J. Manley, J. Aziz, J. L. Padham, and A. M. MacKenzie, "Aging and Factors Related to Running Economy," *Journal of Strength and Conditioning Research* 25 (11) (2011): 2971–2979.

16. S. Melov, M. A. Tarnopolsky, K. Beckman, K. Felkey, and A. Hubbard, "Resistance Exercise Reverses Aging in Human Skeletal Muscle," *PLOS ONE* 2 (5) (2007): e465.

Chapter 5: Training Basics

1. S. Szabo, Y. Tache, and A. Somogyi, "The Legacy of Hans Selye and the Origins of Stress Research: A Retrospective 75 Years After His Landmark Brief 'Letter' to the Editor of *Nature*," *Stress* 15 (5) (2012): 472–478.

2. H. Selye, *Stress Without Distress* (Philadelphia, PA: J. B. Lippincott & Co., 1974).

3. V. B. Issurin, "Generalized Training Effects Induced by Athletic Preparation: A Review," *Journal of Sports Medicine and Physical Fitness* 49 (4) (2009): 333–345.

4. J. Adams and R. Kirkby, "Exercise Dependence: A Review of Its Manifestation, Theory and Measurement," *Sports Medicine, Training and Rehabilitation* 8 (3) (1998): 265–276.

5. D. C. McKenzie, "Markers of Excessive Exercise," *Canadian Journal of Applied Physiology* 24 (1) (1999): 66–73.

6. R. W. Fry, A. R. Morton, and D. Keast, "Periodization and the Prevention of Overtraining," *Canadian Journal of Sport Sciences* 17 (3) (1992): 241–248.

7. N. Berliner, "Anemia in the Elderly," *Transactions of the American Clinical and Climatological Association* 124 (2013): 230–237; D. L. Waters, C. L. Yau, G. D. Montoya, and R. N. Baumgartner, "Serum Sex Hormones, IGF-1, and IGFBP3 Exert a Sexually Dimorphic Effect on Lean Body Mass in Aging," *Journals of Gerontology Series A: Biological Sciences and Medical Sciences* 58 (7) (2003): 648–652; L. Di Luigi, P. Sgrò, V. Fierro, S. Bianchini, G. Battistini, V. Magini, E. A. Jannini, and A. Lenzi, "Prevalence of Undiagnosed Testosterone Deficiency in Aging Athletes: Does Exercise Training Influence the Symptoms of Male Hypogonadism?" *Journal of Sexual Medicine* 7 (7) (2010): 2591–2601.

8. A. C. Hackney, K. P. Hosick, A. Myer, D. A. Rubin, and C. L. Battaglini, "Testosterone Responses to Intensive Interval Versus Steady-State Endurance Exercise," *Journal of Endocrinological Investigation* 35 (11) (2012): 947–950; L. Wideman, J. Y. Weltman, M. L. Hartman, J. D. Veldhuis, and A. Weltman, "Growth Hormone Release During Acute and Chronic Aerobic and Resistance Exercise: Recent Findings," *Sports Medicine* 32 (15) (2002): 987–1004; C. J. Pritzlaff, L. Wideman, J. Y. Weltman, R. D. Abbott, M. E. Gutgesell, M. L. Hartman, J. D. Veldhuis, and A. Weltman, "Impact of Acute Exercise Intensity on Pulsatile Growth Hormone Release in Men," *Journal of Applied Physiology* 87 (2) (1999): 498–504; A. Weltman, J. Y. Weltman, C. P. Roy, L. Wideman, J. Patrie, W. S. Evans, and J. D. Veldhuis, "Growth Hormone Response to Graded Exercise Intensities Is Attenuated and the Gender Difference Abolished in Older Adults," *Journal of Applied Physiology* 100 (5) (2006): 1623–1629.

9. Wideman et al., "Growth Hormone Release"; K. A. Stokes, K. L. Gilbert, G. M. Hall, R. C. Andrews, and D. Thompson, "Different Responses of Selected Hormones to Three Types of Exercise in Young Men," *European Journal of Applied Physiology* 113 (3) (2013): 775–783.

10. C. J. Pritzlaff, L. Wideman, J. Blumer, M. Jensen, R. D. Abbott, G. A. Gaesser, J. D. Veldhuis, and A. Weltman, "Catecholamine Release, Growth Hormone Secretion, and Energy Expenditure During Exercise vs. Recovery in Men," *Journal of Applied Physiology* 89 (3) (2000): 937–946; L. Wideman, J. Y. Weltman, N. Shah, S. Story, J. D. Veldhuis, and A. Weltman, "Effects of Gender on Exercise-Induced Growth Hormone Release," *Journal of Applied Physiology* 87 (3) (1999): 1154–1162.

11. C. Randler, N. Ebenhöh, A. Fischer, S. Höchel, C. Schroff, J. C. Stoll, and C. Vollmer, "Chronotype but Not Sleep Length Is Related to Salivary Testosterone in Young Adult Men," *Psychoneuroendocrinology* 37 (10) (2012): 1740–1744.

12. "Progression of World Record Times for Males," retrieved March 31, 2014, http://www.stat.colostate.edu/~jah/teach/st540/data/mile.info.

13. A. Lucía, J. Hoyos, M. Pérez, and J. L. Chicharro, "Heart Rate and Performance Parameters in Elite Cyclists: A Longitudinal Study," *Medicine and Science in Sports and Exercise* 32 (10) (2000): 1777–1782; A. R. Hoogeveen, "The Effect of Endurance Training on the Ventilator Response to Exercise in Elite Cyclists," *European Journal of Applied Physiology* 82 (1–2) (2000): 45–51.

14. P. Barbeau, O. Serresse, and M. R. Boulay, "Using Maximal and Submaximal Aerobic Variables to Monitor Elite Cyclists During a Season," *Medicine and Science in Sports and Exercise* 25 (9) (1993): 1062–1069.

Chapter 6: Advanced Training

1. I. Tabata, K. Nishimura, M. Kouzaki, Y. Hirai, F. Ogita, M. Miyachi, and K. Yamamoto, "Effects of Moderate-Intensity Endurance and High-Intensity Intermittent Training on Anaerobic Capacity and VO$_2$max," *Medicine and Science in Sports and Exercise* 28 (10) (1996): 1327–1330; P. B. Laursen, C. M. Shing, J. M. Peake, J. S. Coombes, and D. G. Jenkins, "Interval Training Program Optimization in Highly Trained Endurance Cyclists," *Medicine and Science in Sports and Exercise* 34 (11) (2002): 1801–1807; S. Seiler and J. E. Sjursen, "Effect of Work Duration on Physiological and Rating Scale of Perceived Exertion Responses During Self-Paced Interval Training," *Scandinavian Journal of Medicine and Science in Sports* 14 (5) (2004): 318–325; J. Bangsbo, T. P. Gunnarsson, J. Wendell, L. Nybo, and M. Thomassen, "Reduced Volume and Increased Training Intensity Elevate Muscle Na+/K+ Pump {Alpha}2-Subunit Expression as Well as Short- and Long-Term Work Capacity in Humans," *Journal of Applied Physiology* 107 (6) (2009): 1771–1780; J. P. Little, A. Safdar, G. P. Wilkin, M. A. Tarnopolsky, and M. J. Gibala, "A Practical Model of Low-Volume High-Intensity Interval Training Induces Mitochondrial Biogenesis in Human Skeletal Muscle: Potential Mechanisms," *Journal of Physiology* 588, Part 6 (2010): 1011–1022; A. P. Bacon, R. E. Carter, E. A. Ogle, and M. J. Joyner, "VO$_2$max Trainability and High-Intensity Interval Training in Humans: A Meta-Analysis," *PLoS One* 8 (9) (2013): e73182.

2. S. Seiler and K. J. Hetlelid, "The Impact of Rest Duration on Work Intensity and RPE During Interval Training," *Medicine and Science in Sports and Exercise* 37 (9) (2005): 1601–1607.

3. G. P. Millet, R. B. Candau, B. Barbier, T. Busso, J. D. Rouillon, and J. C. Chatard, "Modelling the Transfers of Training Effects on Performance in Elite Triathletes," *International Journal of Sports Medicine* 23 (1) (2002): 55–63.

4. Ibid.; H. Tanaka, "Effects of Cross-Training. Transfer of Training Effects on VO$_2$max Between Cycling, Running and Swimming," *Sports Medicine* 18 (5) (1994): 330–339; J. R. Magel, G. F. Foglia, W. D. McArdle, B. Gutin, G. S. Pechar, and F. I. Katch, "Specificity of Swim Training on Maximum Oxygen Uptake," *Journal of Applied Physiology* 38 (1) (1975): 151–155.

5. E. F. Coyle, "Integration of the Physiological Factors Determining Endurance Performance Ability," *Exercise and Sport Sciences Reviews* 23 (1995): 25–63; L. V. Billat and J. P. Koralsztein, "Significance of the Velocity at VO$_2$max and Time to Exhaustion at this Velocity," *Sports Medicine* 22 (2) (1996): 90–108; V. Billat, V. Binsse, B. Petit, and J. P. Koralsztein, "High Level Runners Are Able to Maintain a VO$_2$ Steady-State Below VO$_2$max in an All-Out Run over Their Critical Velocity," *Archives of Physiology and Biochemistry* 106 (1) (1998): 38–45.

6. L. V. Billat, "Interval Training for Performance: A Scientific and Empirical Practice. Special Recommendations for Middle- and Long-Distance Running. Part II: Anaerobic Interval Training," *Sports Medicine* 31 (2) (2001): 75–90.

7. B. Sjödin, I. Jacobs, and J. Svedenhag, "Changes in Onset of Blood Lactate Accumulation (OBLA) and Muscle Enzymes after Training at OBLA," *European Journal of Applied Physiology* 49 (1) (1982): 45–57.

8. A. W. Midgley, L. R. McNaughton, and M. Wilkinson, "Is There an Optimal Training Intensity for Enhancing the Maximal Oxygen Uptake of Distance Runners?: Empirical Research Findings, Current Opinions, Physiological Rationale and Practical Recommendations," *Sports Medicine* 36 (2) (2006): 117–132.

9. Ibid.

10. J. O. Holloszy and F. W. Booth, "Biochemical Adaptations to Endurance Exercise in Muscle," *Annual Review of Physiology* 38 (1976): 273–291.

11. W. Schmidt, N. Maassen, F. Trost, and D. Böning, "Training-Induced Effects on Blood Volume, Erythrocyte Turnover and Haemoglobin Oxygen Binding Properties," *European Journal of Applied Physiology* 57 (4) (1988): 490–498.

12. B. Mittendorfer and S. Klein, "Physiological Factors that Regulate the Use of Endogenous Fat and Carbohydrate Fuels During Endurance Exercise," *Nutrition Research Reviews* 16 (1) (2003): 97–108; S. Klein, E. F. Coyle, and R. R. Wolfe, "Fat Metabolism During Low-Intensity Exercise in Endurance-Trained and Untrained Men," *American Journal of Physiology* 267 (6), Part 1 (1994): E934–940; M. C. Venables, J. Achten, and A. E. Jeukendrup, "Determinants of Fat Oxidation During Exercise in Healthy Men and Women: A Cross-Sectional Study," *Journal of Applied Physiology* 98 (1) (2005): 160–167.

13. J. S. Skinner and T. M. McLellan, "The Transition from Aerobic to Anaerobic Metabolism," *Research Quarterly for Exercise and Sport* 51 (1) (1980): 234–248; E. Hultman, "Fuel Selection, Muscle Fibre," *Proceedings of the Nutrition Society* 54 (1) (1995): 107–121.

14. W. P. Ebben, A. G. Kindler, K. A. Chirdon, N. C. Jenkins, A. J. Polichnowski, and A. V. Ng, "The Effect of High-Load vs. High-Repetition Training on Endurance Performance," *Journal of Strength and Conditioning Research* 18 (3) (2004): 513–517; J. S. Mikkola, H. K. Rusko, A. T. Nummela, L. M. Paavolainen, and K. Häkkinen, "Concurrent Endurance and Explosive Type Strength Training Increases Activation and Fast Force Production of Leg Extensor Muscles in Endurance Athletes," *Journal of Strength and Conditioning Research* 21 (2) (2007): 613–620; A. Sunde, O. Støren, M. Bjerkaas, M. H. Larsen, J. Hoff, and J. Helgerud, "Maximal Strength Training Improves Cycling Economy in Competitive Cyclists," *Journal of Strength and Conditioning Research* 24 (8) (2010): 2157–2165; P. Aagaard, J. L. Andersen, M. Bennekou, B. Larsson, J. L. Olesen, R. Crameri, S. P. Magnusson, and M. Kjaer, "Effects of Resistance Training on Endurance Capacity and Muscle Fiber Composition in Young Top-Level Cyclists," *Scandinavian Journal of Medicine and Science in Sports* 21 (6) (2011): e298–307; B. R. Rønnestad and I. Mujika, "Optimizing Strength Training for Running and Cycling Endurance Performance: A Review," *Scandinavian Journal of Medicine and Science in Sports* (2013): doi: 10.1111/sms.12104; K. Beattie, I. C. Kenny, M. Lyons, and B. P. Carson, "The Effect of Strength Training on Performance in Endurance Athletes," *Sports Medicine* 44 (6) (2014): 845–865.

15. L. A. Gotshalk, C. C. Loebel, B. C. Nindl, M. Putukian, W. J. Sebastianelli, R. U. Newton, K. Häkkinen, and W. J. Kraemer, "Hormonal Responses of Multiset Versus Single-Set Heavy-Resistance Exercise Protocols," *Canadian Journal of Applied Physiology* 22 (3) (1997): 244–255; K. Goto, M. Nagasawa, O. Yanagisawa, T. Kizuka, N. Ishii, and K. Takamatsu, "Muscular Adaptations to Combinations of High- and Low-Intensity Resistance Exercises," *Journal of Strength and Conditioning Research* 18 (4) (2004): 730–737; J. L. Vingren, W. J. Kraemer, N. A. Ratamess, J. M. Anderson, J. S. Volek, and C. M. Maresh, "Testosterone Physiology in Resistance Exercise and Training: The Up-Stream Regulatory Elements," *Sports Medicine* 40 (12) (2010): 1037–1053; J. P. Ahtiainen, M. Lehti, J. J. Hulmi, W. J. Kraemer, M. Alen, H. Nyman, H. Selänne, A. Pakarinen, J. Komulainen, V. Kovanen, A. A. Mero, and K. Häkkinen, "Recovery after Heavy Resistance Exercise and Skeletal Muscle Androgen Receptor and Insulin-Like Growth Factor-I Isoform Expression in Strength Trained Men," *Journal of Strength and Conditioning Research* 25 (3) (2011): 767–777.

16. H. T. Pitkanen, T. Nykanen, J. Knuutinen, K. Lahti, O. Keinanen, M. Alen, P V. Komi, and A. A. Mero, "Free Amino Acid Pool and Muscle Protein Balance after Resistance Exercise," *Medicine and Science in Sports and Exercise* 35 (5) (2003): 784–792.

17. N. M. Cermak, P. T. Res, L. C. de Groot, W. H. Saris, and L. J. van Loon, "Protein Supplementation Augments the Adaptive Response of Skeletal Muscle to Resistance-Type Exercise Training: A Meta-Analysis," *American Journal of Clinical Nutrition* 96 (6) (2012): 1454–1464.

18. B. Pennings, R. Koopman, M. Beelen, J. M. Senden, W. H. Saris, and L. J. van Loon, "Exercising Before Protein Intake Allows for Greater Use of Dietary Protein-Derived Amino Acids for De Novo Muscle Protein Synthesis in Both Young and Elderly Men," *American Journal of Clinical Nutrition* 93 (2) (2011): 322–331; M. Tieland, M. L. Dirks, N. van der Zwaluw, L. B. Verdijk, O. van de Rest, L. C. de Groot, and L. J. van Loon, "Protein Supplementation Increases Muscle Mass Gain During Prolonged Resistance-Type Exercise Training in Frail Elderly People: A Randomized, Double-Blind, Placebo-Controlled Trial," *Journal of the American Medical Directors Association* 13 (8) (2012): 713–719.

19. K. Häkkinen, M. Alen, W. J. Kraemer, E. Gorostiaga, M. Izquierdo, H. Rusko, J. Mikkola, A. Häkkinen, H. Valkeinen, E. Kaarakainen, S. Romu, V. Erola, J. Ahtiainen, and L. Paavolainen, "Neuromuscular Adaptations During Concurrent Strength and Endurance Training Versus Strength Training," *European Journal of Applied Physiology* 89 (1) (2003): 42–52.

20. G. A. Sforzo and P. R. Touey, "Manipulating Exercise Order Affects Muscular Performance During a Resistance Exercise Training Session," *Journal of Strength and Conditioning Research* 10 (1) (1996): 20–24.

21. D. B. Slarkey, M. A. Welsch, M. L. Pollock, J. E. Graves, W. F. Brechue, and Y. Ishida, "Equivalent Improvement in Strength Following High Intensity, Low and High Volume Training," *Medicine and Science in Sports and Exercise* 26 (5) (1994): S651.

22. J. M. Willardson, "A Brief Review: Factors Affecting the Length of the Rest Interval Between Resistance Exercise Sets," *Journal of Strength and Conditioning Research* 20 (4) (2006): 978–984.

23. J. McDaniel, A. Subudhi, and J. C. Martin, "Torso Stabilization Reduces the Metabolic Cost of Producing Cycling Power," *Canadian Journal of Applied Physiology* 30 (4) (2005): 433–441; D. G. Behm, D. Cappa, and G. A. Power, "Trunk Muscle Activation During Moderate- and High-Intensity Running," *Applied Physiology, Nutrition, and Metabolism* 34 (6) (2009): 1008–1016.

24. T. Hortobágyi, J. A. Houmard, J. R. Stevenson, D. D. Fraser, R. A. Johns, and R. G. Israel, "The Effects of Detraining on Power Athletes," *Medicine and Science in Sports and Exercise* 25 (8) (1993): 929–935.

Chapter 7: Rest and Recovery

1. J. Fell, P. Reaburn, and G. J. Harrison, "Altered Perception and Report of Fatigue and Recovery in Veteran Athletes," *Journal of Sports Medicine and Physical Fitness* 48 (2) (2008): 272–277.

2. J. Fell and D. Williams, "The Effect of Aging on Skeletal-Muscle Recovery from Exercise: Possible Implications for Aging Athletes," *Journal of Aging and Physical Activity* 16 (1) (2008): 97–115.

3. M. Kallinen and A. Markku, "Aging, Physical Activity and Sports Injuries. An Overview of Common Sports Injuries in the Elderly," *Sports Medicine* 20 (1995): 41–52; S. M. Roth, G. F. Martel, F. M. Ivey, J. T. Lemmer, E. J. Metter, B. F. Hurley, and M. A. Rogers, "High-Volume, Heavy Resistance Strength Training and Muscle Damage in Young and Older Women," *Journal of Applied Physiology* 88 (3) (2000): 1112–1118.

4. P. Reaburn, "Poor Use of Post-Exercise Recovery Strategies in Veteran Cyclists: An Australian Study," *Medicine and Science in Sports and Exercise* 45 (5) (2013): S71–74.

5. R. Torres, F. Pinho, J. A. Duarte, and J. M. Cabri, "Effect of Single Bout Versus Repeated Bouts of Stretching on Muscle Recovery Following Eccentric Exercise," *Journal of Science and Medicine in Sport* 16 (6) (2013): 583–588.

6. T. Verde, S. Thomas, and R. J. Shephard, "Potential Markers of Heavy Training in Highly Trained Distance Runners," *British Journal of Sports Medicine* 26 (3) (1992): 167–175.

7. A. E. Jeukendrup, M. K. Hesselink, A. C. Snyder, H. Kuipers, and H. A. Keizer, "Physiological Changes in Male Competitive Cyclists After Two Weeks of Intensified Training," *International Journal of Sports Medicine* 13 (7) (1992): 534–541.

8. V. Vesterinen, K. Häkkinen, E. Hynynen, J. Mikkola, L. Hokka, and A. Nummela, "Heart Rate Variability in Prediction of Individual Adaptation to Endurance Training in Recreational Endurance Runners," *Scandinavian Journal of Medicine and Science in Sports* 23 (2) (2013): 171–180.

9. S. R. Patel, N. T. Ayas, M. R. Malhotra, D. P. White, E. S. Schernhammer, F. E. Speizer, M. J. Stampfer, and F. B. Hu, "A Prospective Study of Sleep Duration and Mortality Risk in Women," *SLEEP* 27 (3) (2004): 440–444; J. E. Ferrie, M. J. Shipley, F. P. Cappuccio, E. Brunner, M. A. Miller, M. Kumari, and M. G. Marmot, "A Prospective Study of Change in Sleep Duration: Associations with Mortality in the Whitehall II Cohort," *SLEEP* 30 (12) (2007): 1659–1666; A. C. Reynolds, J. Dorrian, P. Y. Liu, H. P. A. Van Dongen, G. A. Wittert, L. J. Harmer, and S. Banks, "Impact of Five Nights of Sleep Restriction on Glucose Metabolism, Leptin and Testosterone in Young Adult Men," *PLoS One* 7 (7) (2012): e41218.

10. D. F. Kripke, L. Garfinkel, D. L. Wingard, M. R. Klauber, and M. R. Marler, "Mortality Associated with Sleep Duration and Insomnia," *Archives of General Psychiatry* 59 (2) (2002): 131–136.

11. Ferrie et al., "A Prospective Study of Change in Sleep Duration."

12. Y. He, C. R. Jones, N. Fujiki, Y. Xu, B. Guo, J. L. Holder, Jr., M. J. Rossner, S. Nishino, and Y. H. Fu, "The Transcriptional Repressor DEC2 Regulates Sleep Length in Mammals," *Science* 325 (5942) (2009): 866–870.

13. W. Dement and N. Kleitman, "Cyclic Variations in EEG During Sleep and Their Relation to Eye Movements, Body Motility and Dreaming," *Electroencephalography and Clinical Neurophysiology* 9 (4) (1957): 673–690.

14. R. L. Sack, A. J. Lewy, D. L. Erb, W. M. Vollmer, and C. M. Singer, "Human Melatonin Production Decreases with Age," *Journal of Pineal Research* 3 (4) (1986): 379–388; F. Goldenberg, "Sleep in Normal Aging," *Neurophysiologie Clinique* 21 (4) (1991): 267–279.

15. J. F. Duffy, D. J. Dijk, E. F. Hall, and C. A. Czeisler, "Relationship of Endogenous Circadian Melatonin and Temperature Rhythms to Self-Reported Preference for Morning or Evening Activity in Young and Older People," *Journal of Investigative Medicine* 47 (3) (1999): 141–150; Goldenberg, "Sleep in Normal Aging."

16. H. M. Kravitz, P. A. Ganz, J. Bromberger, L. H. Powell, K. Sutton-Tyrrell, and P. M. Meyer, "Sleep Difficulty in Women at Midlife: A Community Survey of Sleep and the Menopausal Transition," *Menopause* 10 (1) (2003): 19–28.

17. K. Burkhart and J. R. Phelps, "Amber Lenses to Block Blue Light and Improve Sleep: A Randomized Trial," *Chronobiology International* 26 (8) (2009): 1602–1612.

18. A. Vermeulen, "Clinical Review 24: Androgens in the Aging Male," *Journal of Clinical Endocrinology and Metabolism* 73 (2) (1991): 221–224.

19. P. D. Penev, "Association Between Sleep and Morning Testosterone in Older Men," *SLEEP* 30 (4) (2007): 427–432; P. Penev, K. Spiegel, M. L'Hermite-Balériaux, R. Schneider, and E. Van Cauter,

"Relationship Between REM Sleep and Testosterone Secretion in Older Men," *Annales d'Endocrinologie* 64 (2) (2003): 157.

20. A. Mehta and P. C. Hindmarsh, "The Use of Somatropin (Recombinant Growth Hormone) in Children of Short Stature," *Paediatric Drugs* 4 (1) (2002): 37–47.

21. E. Van Cauter, R. Leproult, and L. Plat, "Age-Related Changes in Slow-Wave Sleep and REM Sleep and Relationship with Growth Hormone and Cortisol Levels in Healthy Men," *Journal of the American Medical Association* 284 (7) (2000): 861–868; M. M. Oh, J. W. Kim, M. H. Jin, J. J. Kim, and D. G. Moon, "Influence of Paradoxical Sleep Deprivation and Sleep Recovery on Testosterone Level in Rats of Different Ages," *Asian Journal of Andrology* 14 (2) (2012): 330–334; I. B. Antunes, M. L. Andersen, E. C. Baracat, and S. Tufik, "The Effects of Paradoxical Sleep Deprivation on Estrous Cycles of the Female Rat," *Hormones and Behavior* 49 (4) (2006): 433–440.

22. M. D. de la Calzada, "Modifications in Sleep with Aging," *Revista de Neurologia* 30 (6) (2000): 577–580.

23. Van Cauter, Leproult, and Plat, "Age-Related Changes in Slow-Wave Sleep and REM Sleep."

24. G. Copinschi and E. Van Cauter, "Effects of Aging on Modulation of Hormonal Secretions by Sleep and Circadian Rhythmicity," *Hormone Research* 43 (1–3) (1995): 20–24.

25. M. Ebrecht, J. Hextall, L. G. Kirtley, A. Taylor, M. Dyson, and J. Weinman, "Perceived Stress and Cortisol Levels Predict Speed of Wound Healing in Healthy Male Adults," *Psychoneuroendocrinology* 29 (6) (2004): 798–809.

26. R. P. Knight, Jr., D. S. Kornfeld, G. H. Glaser, and P. K. Bondy, "Effects of Intravenous Hydrocortisone on Electrolytes of Serum and Urine in Man," *Journal of Clinical Endocrinology and Metabolism* 15 (2) (1955): 176–181.

27. I. O. Ebrahim, C. M. Shapiro, A. J. Williams, and P. B. Fenwick, "Alcohol and Sleep I: Effects on Normal Sleep," *Alcoholism Clinical and Experimental Research* 37 (4) (2013): 539–549.

28. G. Howatson, P. G. Bell, J. Tallent, B. Middleton, M. P. McHugh, and J. Ellis, "Effect of Tart Cherry Juice (Prunus Cerasus) on Melatonin Levels and Enhanced Sleep Quality," *European Journal of Nutrition* 51 (8) (2012): 909–916; W. R. Pigeon, M. Carr, C. Gorman, and M. L. Perlis, "Effects of a Tart Cherry Juice Beverage on the Sleep of Older Adults with Insomnia: A Pilot Study," *Journal of Medicinal Food* 13 (3) (2010): 579–583; M. Garrido, D. González-Gómez, M. Lozano, C. Barriga, S. D. Paredes, and A. B. Rodriguez, "A Jerte Valley Cherry Product Provides Beneficial Effects on Sleep Quality: Influence on Aging," *Journal of Nutrition Health and Aging* 17 (6) (2013): 553–560.

29. C. A. Crispim, I. Z. Zimberg, B. G. dos Reis, R. M. Diniz, S. Tufik, and M.T. de Mello, "Relationship Between Food Intake and Sleep Pattern in Healthy Individuals," *Journal of Clinical Sleep Medicine* 7 (6) (2011): 659–664.

30. G. Lindseth, P. Lindseth, and M. Thompson, "Nutritional Effects on Sleep," *Western Journal of Nursing Research* 35 (4) (2013): 497–513.

31. L. V. Thompson, "Skeletal Muscle Adaptations with Age, Inactivity, and Therapeutic Exercise," *Journal of Orthopaedic and Sports Physical Therapy* 32 (2) (2002): 44–57; J. Dorrens and M. J. Rennie, "Effects of Ageing and Human Whole Body and Muscle Protein Turnover," *Scandinavian Journal of Medicine and Science in Sports* 13 (1) (2003): 26–33; W. J. Evans, "Protein Nutrition, Exercise and Aging," *Journal of the American College of Nutrition* 23 (6 Suppl) (2004): 601S–609S; W. W. Campbell, T. A. Trappe, R. R. Wolfe, and W. J. Evans, "The Recommended Dietary Allowance for Protein May Not Be Adequate for Older People to Maintain Skeletal Muscle," *Journals of Gerontology Series A: Biological Sciences and Medical Sciences* 56 (6) (2001): M373–380.

32. E. E. Spangenburg, T. Abraha, T. E. Childs, J. S. Pattison, and F. W. Booth, "Skeletal Muscle IGF-Binding Protein-3 and -5 Expressions Are Age, Muscle, and Load Dependent," *American Journal of Physiology: Endocrinology and Metabolism* 284 (2) (2003): E340–350.

33. P. T. Res, B. Groen, B. Pennings, M. Beelen, G. A. Wallis, A. P. Gijsen, J. M. Senden, and L .J. van Loon, "Protein Ingestion Before Sleep Improves Post-Exercise Overnight Recovery," *Medicine and Science in Sports and Exercise* 44 (8) (2012): 1560–1569.

34. Lindseth, Lindseth, and Thompson, "Nutritional Effects on Sleep."

35. Crispim et al., "Relationship Between Food Intake and Sleep Pattern."

36. S. M. Phillips, "A Brief Review of Critical Processes in Exercise-Induced Muscular Hypertrophy," *Sports Medicine* 44 (S1) (2014): 71–77.

37. Ibid.

38. Ibid.

39. D. Savitha, R. N. Mallikarjuna, and C. Rao, "Effect of Different Musical Tempo on Post-Exercise Recovery in Young Adults," *Indian Journal of Physiology and Pharmacology* 54 (1) (2010): 32–36.

40. A. Barnett, "Using Recovery Modalities Between Training Sessions in Elite Athletes: Does It Help?" *Sports Medicine* 36 (9) (2006): 781–796.

41. K. De Pauw, B. de Geus, B. Roelands, F. Lauwens, J. Verschueren, E. Heyman, and R. R. Meeusen, "Effect of Five Different Recovery Methods on Repeated Cycle Performance," *Medicine and Science in Sports and Exercise* 43 (5) (2011): 890–897.

42. S. Seiler, O. Haugen, and E. Kuffel, "Autonomic Recovery After Exercise in Trained Athletes: Intensity and Duration Effects," *Medicine and Science in Sports and Exercise* 39 (8) (2007): 1366–1373.

43. D. Choi, K. J. Cole, B. H. Goodpaster, W. J. Fink, and D. L. Costill, "Effect of Passive and Active Recovery on the Resynthesis of Muscle Glycogen," *Medicine and Science in Sports and Exercise* 26 (8) (1994): 992–996; S. Ahmaidi, P. Granier, Z. Taoutaou, J. Mercier, H. Dubouchaud, and C. Prefaut, "Effects of Active Recovery on Plasma Lactate and Anaerobic Power Following Repeated Intensive Exercise," *Medicine and Science in Sports and Exercise* 28 (4) (1996): 450–456; A. J. McAinch, M. A. Febbraio, J. M. Parkin, S. Zhao, K. Tangalakis, L. Stojanovska, and M. F. Carey, "Effect of Active Versus Passive Recovery on Metabolism and Performance During Subsequent Exercise," *International Journal of Sport Nutrition and Exercise Metabolism* 14 (2) (2004): 185–196.

44. B. Sperlich, M. Haegele, S. Achtzehn, J. Linville, H. C. Holmberg, and J. Mester, "Different Types of Compression Clothing Do Not Increase Sub-Maximal and Maximal Endurance Performance in Well-Trained Athletes," *Journal of Sports Sciences* 28 (6) (2010): 609–614; D. P. Born, B. Sperlich, and H. C. Holmberg, "Bringing Light into the Dark: Effects of Compression Clothing on Performance and Recovery," *International Journal of Sports Physiology and Performance* 8 (1) (2013): 4–18.

45. R. Duffield, J. Edge, R. Merrells, E. Hawke, M. Barnes, D. Simcock, and N. Gill, "The Effects of Compression Garments on Intermittent Exercise Performance and Recovery on Consecutive Days," *International Journal of Sports Physiology and Performance* 3 (4) (2008): 454–468; V. Davies, K. G. Thompson, and S. M. Cooper, "The Effects of Compression Garments on Recovery," *Journal of Strength and Conditioning Research* 23 (6) (2009): 1786–1794.

46. J. R. Jakeman, C. Byrne, and R. G. Eston, "Lower Limb Compression Garment Improves Recovery from Exercise-Induced Muscle Damage in Young, Active Females," *European Journal of Applied Physiology* 109 (6) (2010): 1137–1144; K. M. de Glanville and M. J. Hamlin, "Positive Effect of Lower Body Compression Garments on Subsequent 40-km Cycling Time Trial Performance," *Journal of Strength and Conditioning Research* 26 (2) (2012): 480–486.

47. M. H. Musani, F. Matta, A. Y. Yaekoub, J. Liang, R. D. Hull, and P. D. Stein, "Venous Compression for Prevention of Postthrombotic Syndrome: A Meta-Analysis," *American Journal of Medicine* 123 (8) (2010): 735–740.

48. A. Wiener, J. Mizrahi, and O. Verbitsky, "Enhancement of Tibialis Anterior Recovery by Intermittent Sequential Pneumatic Compression of the Legs," *Basic and Applied Myology* 11 (2) (2001): 87–90.

49. A. Zelikovski, C. L. Kaye, G. Fink, S. A. Spitzer, and Y. Shapiro, "The Effects of the Modified Intermittent Sequential Pneumatic Device (MISPD) on Exercise Performance Following an Exhaustive Exercise Bout," *British Journal of Sports Medicine* 27 (4) (1993): 255–259.

50. J. Vaile, S. Halson, N. Gill, and B. Dawson, "Effect of Hydrotherapy on Recovery from Fatigue," *International Journal of Sports Medicine* 29 (7) (2008): 539–544; J. Ingram, B. Dawson, C. Goodman, K. Wallman, and J. Beilby, "Effect of Water Immersion Methods on Post-Exercise Recovery from Simulated Team Sport Exercise," *Journal of Science and Medicine in Sport* 12 (3) (2009): 417–421.

51. S. L. Halson, "Does the Time Frame Between Exercise Influence the Effectiveness of Hydrotherapy for Recovery?" *International Journal of Sports Physiology and Performance* 6 (2) (2011): 147–159.

52. T. J. Tucker, D. R. Slivka, J. S. Cuddy, W. S. Hailes, and B. C. Ruby, "Effect of Local Cold Application on Glycogen Recovery," *Journal of Sports Medicine and Physical Fitness* 52 (2) (2012): 158–164; C. Y. Tseng, J. P. Lee, Y. S. Tsai, S. D. Lee, C. L. Kao, T. C. Liu, C. Lai, M. B. Harris, and C. H. Kuo, "Topical Cooling (Icing) Delays Recovery from Eccentric Exercise-Induced Muscle Damage," *Journal of Strength and Conditioning Research* 27 (5) (2013): 1354–1361.

53. G. Z. MacDonald, D. C. Button, E. J. Drinkwater, and D. G. Behm, "Foam Rolling as a Recovery Tool After an Intense Bout of Physical Activity," *Medicine and Science in Sports and Exercise* 46 (1) (2014): 131–142.

54. P. M. Tildus and J. K. Shoemaker, "Effleurage Massage, Muscle Blood Flow and Long-Term Post-Exercise Strength Recovery," *International Journal of Sports Medicine* 16 (7) (1995): 478–483; R. Ogai, M. Yamane, T. Matsumoto, and M. Kosaka, "Effects of Petrissage Massage on Fatigue and Exercise Performance Following Intensive Cycle Pedaling," *British Journal of Sports Medicine* 42 (10) (2008): 834–838.

55. B. Hemmings, M. Smith, J. Graydon, and R. Dyson, "Effects of Massage on Physiological Restoration, Perceived Recovery, and Repeated Sports Performance," *British Journal of Sports Medicine* 34 (2) (2000): 109–114; P. Weerapong, P. A. Hume, and G. S. Kolt, "The Mechanisms of Massage and Effects on Performance, Muscle Recovery and Injury Prevention," *Sports Medicine* 35 (3) (2005): 235–256.

Chapter 8: Body Fat

1. J. C. Seidell and T. L. Visscher, "Body Weight and Weight Change and Their Health Implications for the Elderly," *European Journal of Clinical Nutrition* 54 (Suppl 3) (2000): S33–39; A. B. Newman, J. S. Lee, M. Visser, B. H. Goodpaster, S. B. Kritchevsky, F. A. Tylavsky, M. Nevitt, and T. B. Harris, "Weight Change and the Conservation of Lean Mass in Old Age: The Health, Aging and Body Composition Study," *American Journal of Clinical Nutrition* 82 (4) (2005): 872–878.

2. R. N. Baumgartner, P. M. Stauber, D. McHugh, K. M. Koehler, and P. J. Garry, "Cross-Sectional Age Differences in Body Composition in Persons 60+ Years of Age," *Journals of Gerontology Series A: Biological Sciences and Medical Sciences* 50 (6) (1995): M307–316; D. Gallagher, E. Ruts, M. Visser,

S. Heshka, R. N. Baumgartner, J. Wang, R. N. Pierson, F. X. Pi-Sunyer, and S. B. Heymsfield, "Weight Stability Masks Sarcopenia in Elderly Men and Women," *American Journal of Physiology: Endocrinology and Metabolism* 279 (2) (2000): E366–375.

3. F. S. Celi, "Brown Adipose Tissue—When It Pays to Be Inefficient," *New England Journal of Medicine* 360 (15) (2009): 1553–1556.

4. F. F. Horber, S. A. Kohler, K. Lippuner, and P. Jaeger, "Effect of Regular Physical Training on Age-Associated Alteration of Body Composition in Men," *European Journal of Clinical Investigation* 26 (4) (1996): 279–285.

5. M. Gilliat-Wimberly, M. M. Manore, K. Woolf, P. D. Swan, and S. S. Carroll, "Effects of Habitual Physical Activity on the Resting Metabolic Rates and Body Compositions of Women Aged 35 to 50 Years," *Journal of the American Dietetic Association* 101 (10) (2001): 1181–1188.

6. K. E. Friedl, R. J. Moore, L. E. Martinez-Lopez, J. A. Vogel, E. W. Askew, L. J. Marchitelli, R. W. Hoyt, and C. C. Gordon, "Lower Limit of Body Fat in Healthy Active Men," *Journal of Applied Physiology* 77 (2) (1994): 933–940.

7. Seidell and Visscher, "Body Weight and Weight Change and Their Health Implications for the Elderly"; K. E. Friedl, K. A. Westphal, L. J. Marchitelli, J. F. Patton, W. C. Chumlea, and S. S. Guo, "Evaluation of Anthropometric Equations to Assess Body-Composition Changes in Young Women," *American Journal of Clinical Nutrition* 73 (2) (2001): 268–275; K. A. Shaw, V. K. Srikanth, J. L. Fryer, L. Blizzard, T. Dwyer, and A. J. Venn, "Dual Energy X-Ray Absorptiometry Body Composition and Aging in a Population-Based Older Cohort," *International Journal of Obesity* 31 (2) (2007): 279–284; I. J. Ketel, M. N. Volman, J. C. Seidell, C. D. Stehouwer, J. W. Twisk, and C. B. Lambalk, "Superiority of Skinfold Measurements and Waist over Waist-to-Hip Ratio for Determination of Body Fat Distribution in a Population-Based Cohort of Caucasian Dutch Adults," *European Journal of Endocrinology* 156 (6) (2007): 655–661.

8. A. Vermeulen, S. Goemaere, and J. M. Kaufman, "Testosterone, Body Composition and Aging," *Journal of Endocrinological Investigation* 22 (5 Suppl) (1999): 110–116.

9. Ibid.

10. F. Pasquier, "Diabetes and Cognitive Impairment: How to Evaluate the Cognitive Status?" *Diabetes and Metabolism* 36 (Suppl 3) (2010): S100–105.

11. E. Atlantis, S. A. Martin, M. T. Haren, A. W. Taylor, and G. A. Wittert, "Lifestyle Factors Associated with Age-Related Differences in Body Composition: The Florey Adelaide Male Aging Study," *American Journal of Clinical Nutrition* 88 (1) (2008): 95–104; F. Dela, K. J. Mikines, J. J. Larsen, and H. Galbo, "Training-Induced Enhancement of Insulin Action in Human Skeletal Muscle: The Influence of Aging," *Journals of Gerontology Series A: Biological Sciences and Medical Sciences* 51 (4) (1996): B247–252.

12. Ibid.

13. D. M. Berman, E. M. Rogus, M. J. Busby-Whitehead, L. I. Katzel, and A. P. Goldberg, "Predictors of Adipose Tissue Lipoprotein Lipase in Middle-Aged and Older Men: Relationship to Leptin and Obesity, but not Cardiovascular Fitness," *Metabolism* 48 (2) (1999): 183–189; Atlantis et al., "Lifestyle Factors Associated with Age-Related Differences in Body Composition."

14. M. W. Schwartz, S. C. Woods, D. Porte, Jr., R. J. Seeley, and D. G. Baskin, "Central Nervous System Control of Food Intake," *Nature* 404 (6778) (2000): 661–671.

15. J. Makovey, V. Naganathan, M. Seibel, and P. Sambrook, "Gender Differences in Plasma Ghrelin and Its Relations to Body Composition and Bone—An Opposite-Sex Twin Study," *Clinical Endocrinology* 66 (4) (2007): 530–537.

16. T. Milewicz, J. Krzysiek, A. Janczak-Saif, K. Sztefko, and M. Krzyczkowska-Sendrakowska, "Age, Insulin, SHBG and Sex Steroids Exert Secondary Influence on Plasma Leptin Level in Women," *Endokrynologia Polska* 56 (6) (2005): 883–890.

17. R. Plinta, M. Olszanecka-Glinianowicz, A. Drosdzol-Cop, J. Chudek, and V. Skrzypulec-Plinta, "The Effect of Three-Month Pre-Season Preparatory Period and Short-Term Exercise on Plasma Leptin, Adiponectin, Visfatin, and Ghrelin Levels in Young Female Handball and Basketball Players," *Journal of Endocrinological Investigation* 35 (6) (2012): 595–601; R. Rämson, J. Jürimäe, T. Jürimäe, and J. Mäestu, "The Effect of 4-Week Training Period on Plasma Neuropeptide Y, Leptin and Ghrelin Responses in Male Rowers," *European Journal of Applied Physiology* 112 (5) (2012): 1873–1880.

18. E. Seaborg, "Growing Evidence Links Too Little Sleep to Obesity and Diabetes," *Endocrine News* (2007): 14–15; K. L. Knutson, K. Spiegel, P. Penev, and E. Van Cauter, "The Metabolic Consequences of Sleep Deprivation," *Sleep Medicine Reviews* 11 (3) (2007): 163–178.

19. C. S. Mantzoros, "The Role of Leptin in Human Obesity and Disease: A Review of Current Evidence," *Annals of Internal Medicine* 130 (8) (1999): 671–680.

20. A. V. Nedeltcheva, J. M. Kilkus, J. Imperial, K. Kasza, D. A. Schoeller, and P. D. Penev, "Sleep Curtailment Is Accompanied by Increased Intake of Calories from Snacks," *American Journal of Clinical Nutrition* 89 (1) (2009): 126–133.

21. A. C. Hackney, K. P. Hosick, A. Myer, D. A. Rubin, and C. L. Battaglini, "Testosterone Responses to Intensive Interval Versus Steady-State Endurance Exercise," *Journal of Endocrinological Investigation* 35 (11) (2012): 947–950; K. Sato, M. Iemitsu, K. Matsutani, T. Kurihara, T. Hamaoka, and S. Fujita, "Resistance Training Restores Muscle Sex Steroid Hormone Steroidogenesis in Older Men," *Federation of American Societies for Experimental Biology Journal* 28 (4) (2014): 1891–1897.

22. S. K. Das, C. H. Gilhooly, J. K. Golden, A. G. Pittas, P. J. Fuss, R. A. Cheatham, S. Tyler, M. Tsay, M. A. McCrory, A. H. Lichtenstein, G. E. Dallal, C. Dutta, M. V. Bhapkar, J. P. Delany, E. Saltzman, and S. B. Roberts, "Long-Term Effects of 2 Energy-Restricted Diets Differing in Glycemic Load on Dietary Adherence, Body Composition, and Metabolism in CALERIE: A 1-y Randomized Controlled Trial," *American Journal of Clinical Nutrition* 85 (4) (2007): 1023–1030.

23. C. H. Gilhooly, S. K. Das, J. K. Golden, M. A. McCrory, G. E. Dallal, E. Saltzman, F. M. Kramer, and S. B. Roberts, "Food Cravings and Energy Regulation: The Characteristics of Craved Foods and Their Relationship with Eating Behaviors and Weight Change During 6 Months of Dietary Energy Restriction," *International Journal of Obesity* 31 (12) (2007): 1849–1858.

24. D. E. Thomas, E. J. Elliott, and L. Baur, "Low Glycaemic Index or Low Glycaemic Load Diets for Overweight and Obesity," *Cochrane Database of Systematic Reviews* 18 (3) (2007): CD005105; A. Esfahani, J. M. Wong, A. Mirrahimi, C. R. Villa, and C. W. Kendall, "The Application of the Glycemic Index and Glycemic Load in Weight Loss: A Review of the Clinical Evidence," *International Union of Biochemistry and Molecular Biology Life* 63 (1) (2011): 7–13.

25. F. S. Atkinson, K. Foster-Powell, and J. C. Brand-Miller, "International Tables of Glycemic Index and Glycemic Load Values: 2008," *Diabetes Care* 31 (12) (2008): 2281–2283.

26. D. Paddon-Jones and H. Leidy, "Dietary Protein and Muscle in Older Persons," *Current Opinion in Clinical Nutrition and Metabolic Care* 17 (1) (2014): 5–11.

27. P. Britten, L. E. Cleveland, K. L. Koegel, K. J. Kuczynski, and S. M. Nickols-Richardson, "Updated US Department of Agriculture Food Patterns Meet Goals of the 2010 Dietary Guidelines," *Journal of the Academy of Nutrition and Dietetics* 112 (10) (2012): 1648–1655.

28. R. Elango, M. A. Humayun, R. O. Ball, and P. B. Pencharz, "Evidence that Protein Requirements Have Been Significantly Underestimated," *Current Opinion in Clinical Nutrition and Metabolic*

Care 13 (1) (2010): 52–57; J. Bauer, G. Biolo, T. Cederholm, M. Cesari, A. J. Cruz-Jentoft, J. E. Morley, S. Phillips, C. Sieber, P. Stehle, D. Teta, R. Visvanathan, E. Volpi, and Y. Boirie, "Evidence-Based Recommendations for Optimal Dietary Protein Intake in Older People: A Position Paper from the PROT-AGE Study Group," *Journal of the American Medical Directors Association* 14 (8) (2013): 542–559.

29. M. M. Mamerow, J. A. Mettler, K. L. English, S. L. Casperson, E. Arentson-Lantz, M. Sheffield-Moore, D. K. Layman, and D. Paddon-Jones, "Dietary Protein Distribution Positively Influences 24-h Muscle Protein Synthesis in Healthy Adults," *Journal of Nutrition* 144 (6) (2014): 876–880.

30. R. K. Krishnan, W. J. Evans, and J. P. Kirwan, "Impaired Substrate Oxidation in Healthy Elderly Men After Eccentric Exercise," *Journal of Applied Physiology* 94 (2) (2003): 716–723.

31. S. H. Holt, J. C. Miller, P. Petocz, and E. Farmakalidis, "A Satiety Index of Common Foods," *European Journal of Clinical Nutrition* 49 (9) (1995): 675–690.

32. T. L. Halton and F. B. Hu, "The Effects of High Protein Diets on Thermogenesis, Satiety and Weight Loss: A Critical Review," *Journal of the American College of Nutrition* 23 (5) (2004): 373–385; R. F. Kushner and B. Doerfler, "Low-Carbohydrate, High-Protein Diets Revisited," *Current Opinion in Gastroenterology* 24 (2) (2008): 198–203; B. J. Brehm and D. A. D'Alessio, "Benefits of High-Protein Weight Loss Diets: Enough Evidence for Practice?" *Current Opinion in Endocrinology, Diabetes and Obesity* 15 (5) (2008): 416–421.

33. M. A. Singh, "Combined Exercise and Dietary Intervention to Optimize Body Composition in Aging," *Annals of the New York Academy of Sciences* 854 (1998): 378–393; W. J. Evans, "Protein Nutrition, Exercise and Aging," *Journal of the American College of Nutrition* 23 (6 Suppl) (2004): 601S-609S; W. W. Campbell, "Synergistic Use of Higher-Protein Diets or Nutritional Supplements with Resistance Training to Counter Sarcopenia," *Nutrition Reviews* 65 (9) (2007): 416–422; R. M. Daly, S. L. O'Connell, N. L. Mundell, C. A. Grimes, D. W. Dunstan, and C. A. Nowson, "Protein-Enriched Diet, with the Use of Lean Red Meat, Combined with Progressive Resistance Training Enhances Lean Tissue Mass and Muscle Strength and Reduces Circulating IL-6 Concentrations in Elderly Women: A Cluster Randomized Controlled Trial," *American Journal of Clinical Nutrition* 99 (4) (2014): 899–910.

34. N. M. Cermak, P. T. Res, L. C. de Groot, W. H. Saris, and L. J. van Loon, "Protein Supplementation Augments the Adaptive Response of Skeletal Muscle to Resistance-Type Exercise Training: A Meta-Analysis," *American Journal of Clinical Nutrition* 96 (6) (2012): 1454–1464; K. D. Tipton and S. M. Phillips, "Dietary Protein for Muscle Hypertrophy," *Nestlé Nutrition Institute Workshop Series* 76 (2013): 73–84; D. M. Camera, D. W. West, S. M. Phillips, T. Rerecich, T. Stellingwerff, J. A. Hawley, and V. G. Coffey, "Protein Ingestion Increases Myofibrillar Protein Synthesis After Concurrent Exercise," *Medicine and Science in Sports and Exercise* (2014), doi:10.1249/MSS.0000000000000390.

35. R. S. Surwit, M. N. Feinglos, J. Rodin, A. Sutherland, A. E. Petro, E. C. Opara, C. M. Kuhn, and M. Rebuffé-Scrive, "Differential Effects of Fat and Sucrose on the Development of Obesity and Diabetes in C57BL/6J and A/J Mice," *Metabolism* 44 (5) (1995): 645–651; A. Shapiro, N. Tümer, Y. Gao, K. Y. Cheng, and P. J. Scarpace, "Prevention and Reversal of Diet-Induced Leptin Resistance with a Sugar-Free Diet Despite High Fat Content," *British Journal of Nutrition* 106 (3) (2011): 390–397.

36. M. L. Pollock, C. Foster, D. Knapp, J. L. Rod, and D. H. Schmidt, "Effect of Age and Training on Aerobic Capacity and Body Composition of Master Athletes," *Journal of Applied Physiology* 62 (2) (1987): 725–731.

37. A. Tremblay, J. A. Simoneau, and C. Bouchard, "Impact of Exercise Intensity on Body Fatness and Skeletal Muscle Metabolism," *Metabolism* 43 (7) (1994): 814–818.

38. T. Douchi, S. Yamamoto, T. Oki, K. Maruta, R. Kuwahata, H. Yamasaki, and Y. Nagata, "The Effects of Physical Exercise on Body Fat Distribution and Bone Mineral Density in Postmenopausal

Women," *Maturitas* 35 (1) (2000): 25–30; T. Douchi, T. Matsuo, H. Uto, T. Kuwahata, T. Oki, and Y. Nagata, "Lean Body Mass and Bone Mineral Density in Physically Exercising Postmenopausal Women," *Maturitas* 45 (3) (2003): 185–190.

39. O. L. Svendsen, C. Hassager, and C. Christiansen, "Age- and Menopause-Associated Variations in Body Composition and Fat Distribution in Healthy Women as Measured by Dual-Energy X-Ray Absorptiometry," *Metabolism* 44 (3) (1995): 369–373; T. Douchi, S. Kosha, H. Uto, T. Oki, M. Nakae, N. Yoshimitsu, and Y. Nagata, "Precedence of Bone Loss over Changes in Body Composition and Body Fat Distribution Within a Few Years After Menopause," *Maturitas* 46 (2) (2003): 133–138.

40. T. Douchi, S. Yamamoto, N. Yoshimitsu, T. Andoh, T. Matsuo, and Y. Nagata, "Relative Contribution of Aging and Menopause to Changes in Lean and Fat Mass in Segmental Regions," *Maturitas* 42 (4) (2002): 301–306; T. Douchi, Y. Yonehara, Y. Kawamura, A. Kuwahata, T. Kuwahata, and I. Iwamoto, "Difference in Segmental Lean and Fat Mass Components Between Pre- and Postmenopausal Women," *Menopause* 14 (5) (2007): 875–878.

41. E. T. Poehlman and A. Tchernof, "Traversing the Menopause: Changes in Energy Expenditure and Body Composition," *Coronary Artery Disease* 9 (12) (1998): 799–803; E. T. Poehlman, M. J. Toth, and A. W. Gardner, "Changes in Energy Balance and Body Composition at Menopause: A Controlled Longitudinal Study," *Annals of Internal Medicine* 123 (9) (1995): 673–675; A. Tchernof and E. T. Poehlman, "Effects of the Menopause Transition on Body Fatness and Body Fat Distribution," *Obesity Research* 6 (3) (1998): 246–254; H. Ijuin, T. Douchi, T. Oki, K. Maruta, and Y. Nagata, "The Contribution of Menopause to Changes in Body-Fat Distribution," *Journal of Obstetrics and Gynaecology Research* 25 (5) (1999): 367–372; M. J. Toth, A. Tchernof, C. K. Sites, and E. T. Poehlman, "Menopause-Related Changes in Body Fat Distribution," *Annals of the New York Academy of Sciences* 904 (2000): 502–506.

42. J. M. Hagberg, J. M. Zmuda, S. D. McCole, K. S. Rodgers, K. R. Wilund, and G. E. Moore, "Determinants of Body Composition in Postmenopausal Women," *Journals of Gerontology Series A: Biological Sciences and Medical Sciences* 55 (10) (2000): M607–612.

43. T. N. Waldman, "Menopause: When Hormone Replacement Therapy Is Not an Option. Part I," *Journal of Women's Health* 7 (5) (1998): 559–565; A. Lukes, "Evolving Issues in the Clinical and Managed Care Settings on the Management of Menopause Following the Women's Health Initiative," *Journal of Managed Care Pharmacy* 14 (3 Suppl) (2008): 7–13.

44. W. S. Leslie, C. R. Hankey, and M. E. Lean, "Weight Gain as an Adverse Effect of Some Commonly Prescribed Drugs: A Systematic Review," *Quarterly Journal of Medicine* 100 (7) (2007): 395–404.

45. H. Pijl and A. E. Meinders, "Bodyweight Change as an Adverse Effect of Drug Treatment: Mechanisms and Management," *Drug Safety* 14 (5) (1996): 329–342; L. J. Cheskin, S. J. Bartlett, R. Zayas, C. H. Twilley, D. B. Allison, and C. Contoreggi, "Prescription Medications: A Modifiable Contributor to Obesity," *Southern Medical Journal* 92 (9) (1999): 898–904; S. K. Kulkarni and G. Kaur, "Pharmacodynamics of Drug-Induced Weight Gain," *Drugs Today* 37 (8) (2001): 559–571; L. J. Aronne and K. R. Segal, "Weight Gain in the Treatment of Mood Disorders," *Journal of Clinical Psychiatry* 64 (Suppl 8) (2003): 22–29; M. Malone, "Medications Associated with Weight Gain," *Annals of Pharmacotherapy* 39 (12) (2005): 2046–2055; R. Ness-Abramof and C. M. Apovian, "Drug-Induced Weight Gain," *Drugs Today* 41 (8) (2005): 547–555; D. I. Brixner, Q. Said, P. K. Corey-Lisle, A. V. Tuomari, G. J. L'italien, W. Stockdale, and G. M. Oderda, "Naturalistic Impact of Second-Generation Antipsychotics on Weight Gain," *Annals of Pharmacotherapy* 40 (4) (2006): 626–632; "Prescription Meds Can Put On Unwanted Pounds," http://www.drugs.com/news/meds-can-put-unwanted-pounds-36772.html.

46. W. D. McArdle, F. I. Katch, and V. L. Katch, *Essentials of Exercise Physiology*, 4th ed. (Baltimore, MD: Williams & Wilkins, 1996): 396–403.

About the Contributors

MARK ALLEN is a six-time Hawaii Ironman World Champion. His first six attempts to win the race ended in defeat, but each helped galvanize his commitment to achieving his dream of becoming champion. Finally, in 1989, on his seventh try, Mark won the first of what many consider to be the toughest one-day sporting event in the world.

Over the course of a 15-year racing career, Mark maintained a 90 percent average in top-three finishes and won 66 of the 96 races in which he competed. He was named "Triathlete of the Year" six times by *Triathlete* magazine, and in 1997 *Outside* magazine called him "The World's Fittest Man." In November 2012 Mark was voted "The Greatest Endurance Athlete of All Time" in a worldwide poll conducted by ESPN. He retired from racing in 1996.

Today Mark shares his stories of Ironman racing with top corporate audiences throughout the world; has a triathlon coaching service used in over 50 countries; is the coauthor with Brant Secunda of the award-winning book *Fit Soul, Fit Body: 9 Keys to a Healthier, Happier You*; and has recently published a new book, *The Art of Competition*.

GALE BERNHARDT has instructed or coached athletes since 1974. Her first Olympic experience was serving as the personal coach for an individual cyclist at the 2000 Sydney Olympic Games. Her athlete won the 2000 USA Cycling Pro National Championship race, thus securing a spot on the 2000 Olympic team.

In 2003, Gale was selected by USA Triathlon to serve as the Pan American Games coach for the men's and women's teams. In 2004 Gale was selected as coach of both the men's and women's triathlon teams for the Athens Olympic Games.

Gale has a BS degree from Colorado State University and is certified as a Level I Coach by USA Cycling and a Level III Coach by USA Triathlon, the highest certifications available in both sports. She served on the USA Triathlon National Coaching Committee from 2000 to 2006. She served as the committee chair-elect immediately after joining the committee and went on to serve as the chairperson for five consecutive years.

Gale's success and experience led to her being selected as a World Cup Coach for the International Triathlon Union (ITU) Sport Development squad. In addition to her work for the ITU, Gale has served as a presenter at coaching clinics and corporate team championships.

AMBY BURFOOT is 68; he began running in college, where his roommate was Bill Rodgers, who later became one of America's all-time best marathoners. Burfoot won the 1968 Boston Marathon. An injury resulting from a steeplechase race in a collegiate track meet later that spring prevented him from being fully prepared for that year's Olympic Trials marathon, but in the Fukuoka Marathon in Japan in December 1968, Burfoot ran a personal best of 2:14:29, which was only 1 second from the American marathon record at the time. At Burfoot's peak, his training often included weeks of 100 to 140 miles. Later in life, after retiring from international competition, Burfoot became a running journalist and author. He was editor in chief of *Runner's World* for many years and now serves as the magazine's editor at large.

LARRY CRESWELL, MD, is a heart surgeon and faculty member at the University of Mississippi School of Medicine in Jackson. He is a graduate of the University of Pennsylvania and the Johns Hopkins University School of Medicine. His clinical practice focuses on adult heart surgery—bypass surgery, heart valve repair/replacement, aortic surgery, and heart transplantation. Larry is an avid triathlete and open-water swimmer and, at 51, a veteran athlete himself. He has an interest in athletes and all forms of heart disease, with a particular emphasis on the heart problems of endurance athletes. Larry recently led a USA Triathlon medical panel review of race-related fatalities and was recognized for his contributions as the USA Triathlon Volunteer of the Year.

JOHN HOWARD was a three-time Olympic cyclist (1968, 1972, and 1976) who also set a land speed record of 152.2 mph in 1985 on Utah's Bonneville Salt Flats. He dominated U.S. road cycling in the 1970s, winning 18 U.S. National Cycling Championships at the peak of his racing career. Howard also captured the first two editions of the Red Zinger Bicycle Classic stage race in Colorado in 1975 and 1976. In 1971 he won the gold medal in the Pan American Games road cycling race. In 1982 he was one of four competitors in the inaugural Race Across America (RAAM), eventually finishing second. In 1987, he set the world record for the 24-hour cycling ultramarathon (539 miles). His dominance as an endurance athlete went beyond cycling. In 1981 he won the Ironman Triathlon World Championship in Hawaii. He also held the American Canoe Association's world record for 24 hours (104.6 miles).

TIM NOAKES, OMS, MBChB, MD, DSc, PhD (hc), is a professor of exercise and sports science in South Africa. He has run more than 70 marathons and ultramarathons and is the author of the best-selling running book *Lore of Running*. He also wrote *Waterlogged*; *Challenging Beliefs*; and, recently, *The Real Meal Revolution*. In 1980 he started the sports science department at the University of Cape Town, where he still teaches. Among a vast array of sport science topics, he is a recognized authority on hyponatremia in endurance sports, the central-governor theory of exercise fatigue and nutrition.

NED OVEREND has raced mountain bikes for three decades. In that time he has collected the titles of UCI (Union Cycliste Internationale) Mountain Bike Cross-Country World Champion (the first ever in 1990), U.S. National Cross-Country Champion (six times), and XTERRA Triathlon World Champion (twice). Recently, at the age of 55, he became the 2010 Single Speed National Champion.

Ned is an inductee of the Mountain Bike Hall of Fame, the U.S. Bicycling Hall of Fame, and the XTERRA Hall of Fame. His contributions to trail advocacy in his hometown of Durango, Colorado, have been recognized with the naming of Overend Mountain Park. He is a board member of Bicycle Colorado and an honorary board member of the International Mountain Bicycling Association and works at Specialized Bicycles in sports marketing and product development.

JOHN POST, MD, is an orthopedic surgeon in Charlottesville, Virginia, with 30 years of triathlon experience. He is a Naval Academy graduate and was a helicopter pilot in Vietnam. His practice is centered on diseases of the knee and shoulder and physician education. He is a six-time Ironman Hawaii finisher, has completed the Around Manhattan Swimming Marathon, and is married with three children.

ANDREW L. PRUITT, EdD, is an internationally known athletic trainer, physician assistant, and teacher. Pruitt is director of the Boulder Center for Sports Medicine (BCSM) in Boulder, Colorado. He is one of the world's foremost experts on bike fit and cycling injuries. Pruitt headed the U.S. Cycling Federation's sports medicine program for many years, including four World Championships. He was the chief medical officer for U.S. Cycling at the 1996 Olympics in Atlanta and helped design medical coverage for the Atlanta cycling venues on a model he developed as medical director of the Tour DuPont. Pruitt is the recognized leader in computerized cycling gait analysis, a technique that uses three-dimensional computer technology to determine perfect bike fit for any rider (a service available at the BCSM).

LISA RAINSBERGER (formerly Weidenbach) is the last American woman to have won the Boston Marathon, doing so in a time of 2:34:06 in 1985. She has four marathon times in the top-100 all-time-best performances by U.S. women. Her personal best time was 2:28:15. She is a member of the University of Michigan Track and Field and Road Runners Club of America Halls of Fame. Rainsberger won competitions as a swimmer in the individual medley, qualifying for the 1980 U.S. Olympic Swim Trials, and later competed on scholarship as an All-American swimmer at the University of Michigan. In college she was also a two-time All-American in track and cross country. In 1984 she ran the inaugural women's U.S. Olympic marathon trials, finishing fourth and just missing a spot in that year's Olympic Games. Rainsberger won the Chicago Marathon in back-to-back years in 1988 (2:29:17) and 1989 (2:28:15), something no American woman has done since. She now focuses on her family and her coaching business, Training Goals (www.traininggoals.com).

Index

About the Author

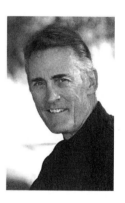

Joe Friel is the cofounder of TrainingPeaks.com and TrainingBible Coaching. With a master of science degree in exercise science, he has coached and trained endurance athletes since 1980. His clients have included road cyclists, mountain bikers, triathletes, runners, rowers, and endurance horse racers. He has coached athletes of all ages and abilities from novice to elite, both amateurs and professionals. The list includes an Ironman Triathlon winner, USA and foreign national champions, world championship competitors, and an Olympian.

Joe is the author of the following books: *The Cyclist's Training Bible*, *The Triathlete's Training Bible*, *The Mountain Biker's Training Bible*, *Cycling Past 50*, *Going Long* (coauthor), *The Paleo Diet for Athletes* (coauthor), *Your First Triathlon*, *Your Best Triathlon*, *The Power Meter Handbook*, *Precision Heart Rate Training* (contributor), *Total Heart Rate Training*, and *Triathlon Science* (coeditor). He helped found the USA Triathlon National Coaching Commission and served two terms as chairman.

He has been a columnist for *Inside Triathlon, VeloNews,* and more than 200 other magazines and frequently writes articles for international magazines and websites. His opinions on matters related to training for endurance sports are widely sought and have been featured in such publications as *Runner's World, Outside, Triathlete, Women's Sports & Fitness, Men's Fitness, Men's Health, American Health, Masters Sports, Walking, Bicycling,* the *New York Times,* and *Vogue.*

He conducts seminars and camps on training and racing for endurance athletes and coaches in Asia, Europe, North and South America, and the Pacific region. He also provides consulting services to corporations in the fitness industry and to national governing bodies.

As an age-group competitor, he is a former Colorado State Masters Triathlon Champion and a Rocky Mountain region and Southwest region duathlon age-group champion. He has been named to several All-American teams and has represented the United States at world championships. He now competes in USA Cycling bike races and time trials.

Joe may be contacted through his blog at joefrielsblog.com.